CARB CYCLING FOR WOMEN OVER 50

EFFECTIVE GUIDE TO NUTRITIOUS WELLBEING WITH HIGH, MODERATE AND LOW CARB DAYS FOR SENIOR WOMEN

ANITA MICHEL

ISBN: 9798325491139

Cover design by: Art Painter
Library of Congress Control Number: 2018675309
Printed in the United States of America

This book is dedicated to my Mom, Mrs michel
Your belief in me fueled every word, and your patience in moments of doubt kept
the flame of creativity alive. Thank you for being the wind beneath my wings,
propelling me to reach new heights. This work is as much yours as it is mine

CONTENTS

INTRODUCTION

Welcome to "Carb Cycling for Women Over 50" – your go-to guide for unlocking the secrets of nutrition tailored specifically for women navigating the vibrant years beyond 50. If you're flipping through these pages, chances are you've already embraced the wisdom that comes with age and are keen on optimizing your well-being. Well, you're in the right place!

As we gracefully age, our bodies undergo various changes – hormonal fluctuations, metabolic shifts, and lifestyle adjustments. One thing that remains constant, though, is the significance of a well-balanced and personalized nutrition plan. Enter carb cycling – a dynamic approach to fueling your body with the right nutrients at the right times.

But why the focus on women over 50? Because, my friend, this is a unique chapter in your life where wisdom meets vitality, and we want to ensure you're thriving, not just surviving. We understand that the cookie-cutter diets of yesteryears might not cut it anymore. It's time to tailor your nutrition to fit the fabulous woman you've become.

Now, let's get real for a moment. We get it – the world of nutrition can be overwhelming. Fad diets, conflicting advice, and an abundance of information that seems to change with every passing season. It's enough to make your head spin! That's where "Carb Cycling for women over 50 steps in as your reliable companion on this journey to wellness.

So, what exactly is carb cycling, and why should it be on your radar? Great questions! Carb cycling is not a one-size-fits-all solution; it's a flexible and sustainable approach to eating that takes into account your individual needs, activity levels, and, most importantly, your age. In the following pages, we'll delve into the science behind carb cycling, breaking it down into digestible bits (pun intended) so you can easily grasp how it can become your secret weapon for feeling fantastic at 50 and beyond.

As women over 50, we've earned our stripes – a lifetime of experiences, accomplishments, and maybe a few challenges that made us stronger. But with this badge of honor comes the responsibility to prioritize our health and well-being. The truth is, we can't rely on the nutrition plans of our younger days. Our bodies demand a different kind of attention, and that's where carb cycling steps in to meet those demands.

This book is not about deprivation, counting every calorie, or spending endless hours in the gym. Instead, it's about empowering you with the knowledge to make informed choices about the foods you eat and when you eat them. It's about embracing a lifestyle that allows you to savor the flavors of life while ensuring your body gets the nourishment it deserves.

Throughout these pages, you'll find practical advice, customizable meal plans, and real-life stories from women who, like you, are navigating the exciting journey of life over 50. We'll guide you through the science, help you design a carb cycling plan that suits your lifestyle, and address common challenges that might pop up along the way.

Consider this book your personalized roadmap to a healthier, more vibrant you. Whether you're a fitness enthusiast looking to optimize your workouts, someone aiming to manage weight, or simply a woman who wants to feel her best, "Carb Cycling for Women Over 50" is your trusted companion.   So, grab a cozy blanket, a cup of your favorite tea, and let's embark on this journey together – because your best years are yet to come, and we're here to make sure they're filled with health, happiness, and the perfect balance of carbs!

CHAPTER 1: FOUNDATIONS OF CARB CYCLING

Basic of Micronutrient

In the ever-evolving landscape of nutrition, the term "macronutrients" often gets thrown around, but what do they really mean, and why should we care? Well, dear reader, let's dive into the fundamentals.

Macronutrients, or macros for short, are the nutrients our bodies require in relatively large quantities to function optimally. There are three primary players in the macronutrient game: carbohydrates, proteins, and fats. Each plays a crucial role in supporting various bodily functions, and understanding their significance is key to embarking on a successful carb cycling journey.

Carbohydrates: Often misunderstood and unfairly demonized, carbohydrates are the body's preferred source of energy. Found in foods like grains, fruits, and vegetables, carbs are broken down into glucose, providing fuel for our cells and energy for our daily activities. However, not all carbs are created equal. The distinction between simple carbohydrates (sugars) and complex carbohydrates (fiber-rich) is vital in crafting a carb cycling plan that optimally supports your body.

Proteins: Known as the building blocks of life, proteins are essential for repairing and building tissues. Found in meat, fish, eggs, and plant-based sources like beans and tofu, proteins are integral to maintaining muscle mass, supporting immune function, and keeping our skin, hair, and nails healthy. When it comes to carb cycling, understanding how protein intake can be adjusted based on activity levels and goals is key to achieving the desired results.

Fats: Contrary to outdated beliefs, fats are not the enemy. In fact, they play a crucial role in hormone production, nutrient absorption, and overall cellular function. Avocados, nuts, seeds, and olive oil are excellent sources of healthy fats. Balancing fat intake becomes crucial in a carb cycling approach, as it contributes to sustained energy levels and helps regulate appetite.

Understanding the interplay of these macronutrients lays the foundation for creating a carb cycling plan that aligns with your body's needs. It's not about vilifying any particular macronutrient but rather finding the right balance that promotes overall health and supports your individual goals.

How Carbohydrates Affect the Body

Now that we've brushed up on the basics of macronutrients, let's zoom in on the star of the show – carbohydrates. These energy-packed compounds are the body's primary fuel source, but the key lies in understanding how different types of carbs impact our physiology.

Simple Carbohydrates: Think of these as the quick-burning fuel for your body. Found in sugary snacks, sodas, and processed foods, simple carbs cause a rapid spike in blood sugar levels, followed by a crash. While they can provide a quick energy boost, relying on them can lead to energy fluctuations and cravings, which is why they have a limited role in carb cycling.

Complex Carbohydrates: The heroes of sustained energy come in the form of complex carbs. Found in whole grains, vegetables, and legumes, these carbs are rich in fiber, which slows down the absorption of glucose. This slow and steady release of energy helps maintain stable blood sugar levels, providing a consistent fuel source without the rollercoaster of highs and lows.

Impact on Insulin: Carbohydrates, especially in the form of simple sugars, can affect insulin levels in the body. Insulin plays a crucial role in regulating blood sugar, and understanding how different carb sources influence insulin release is pivotal in crafting a carb cycling plan. By strategically managing carbohydrate intake, we can optimize insulin sensitivity, promoting better energy utilization and fat metabolism. In the context of carb cycling for women over 50, this nuanced understanding of carbohydrates becomes even more critical. As our bodies undergo hormonal changes with age, the way we process and utilize carbs may shift. Tailoring our carb intake to support these changes is a key aspect of optimizing nutrition for this specific demographic.

I mportance of Tailoring Nutrition to Age and Gender
Here's a truth bomb – a nutrition plan that worked wonders in your 20s might not yield the same results in your 50s. As we age, our bodies undergo various changes, and these changes necessitate a customized approach to nutrition. Furthermore, the impact of age is not uniform across genders; men and women may experience different nutritional needs and challenges.

Hormonal Changes: For women over 50, hormonal fluctuations, particularly during menopause, can influence metabolism and body composition. Estrogen levels decrease, affecting how the body stores and utilizes fat. Understanding these hormonal shifts is crucial in adapting carb cycling to support hormonal balance and mitigate potential challenges like weight gain and muscle loss.

Metabolic Rate: Age-related changes in metabolism are inevitable. The basal metabolic rate (BMR) tends to decrease with age, meaning our bodies burn fewer calories at rest. Tailoring carb intake to accommodate these metabolic changes is essential for preventing unwanted weight gain and sustaining energy levels.

Bone Health: Women, in particular, face a higher risk of osteoporosis as they age. Adequate nutrition, including essential vitamins and minerals, becomes paramount in supporting bone health. Tailoring carb cycling to include nutrient-dense foods that promote bone strength is a proactive step in

mitigating age related bone issues.

Individualized Goals: While age sets a general framework, individual factors play a

significant role in shaping nutritional needs. Factors such as activity level, pre-existing health conditions, and personal fitness goals all contribute to the complexity of designing an effective carb cycling plan. Tailoring nutrition to the unique combination of age and individual circumstances ensure a plan that is not only effective but also sustainable in the long run.

In the world of nutrition, one size does not fit all, and the same holds true for carb cycling. Recognizing the nuanced relationship between age, gender, and nutrition sets the stage for a tailored approach that empowers women over 50 to navigate this exciting chapter of life with vitality and optimal wellbeing.

It's not just about what you eat; it's about what your body specifically needs at this stage in the journey.

CHAPTER 2: THE SCIENCE BEHIND CARB CYCLING

Metabolic Changes in Women Over 50

The journey through the golden years brings with it a host of changes, and perhaps one of the most notable is the inevitable slowing down of metabolism. Understanding these metabolic shifts is essential when delving into the world of carb cycling, especially for women over 50.

Basal Metabolic Rate (BMR): At the core of metabolic changes is the Basal Metabolic Rate, the number of calories the body requires at rest. In our 50s, BMR tends to decrease gradually. This means that the body burns fewer calories during periods of inactivity, making weight management more challenging. Carb cycling becomes a strategic tool to navigate this shift, ensuring that energy intake aligns with the body's evolving metabolic needs.

Muscle Mass and Metabolism: Another factor influencing metabolism is the natural decline in muscle mass that accompanies aging, known as sarcopenia. Muscle tissue is metabolically active, meaning it burns more calories than fat even at rest. As muscle mass diminishes, so does the body's calorie-burning capacity. Carb cycling, when structured with attention to protein intake and resistance training, can help preserve muscle mass, thus mitigating the impact of age-related metabolic changes.

Nutrient Partitioning: Metabolic changes also affect how the body partitions nutrients, particularly carbohydrates. In the carb cycling context, understanding how the body utilizes and stores carbs is crucial. With age, there is a tendency for the body to become less efficient in using carbohydrates for energy, leading to potential excess storage as fat. By strategically adjusting carbohydrate intake through carb cycling, women over 50 can optimize nutrient utilization and manage body composition effectively.

Navigating metabolic changes isn't about resisting the natural course of aging; it's about adapting our approach to nutrition to support our bodies through each phase. Carb cycling emerges as a dynamic strategy to harmonize with these changes, ensuring that our metabolic machinery continues to function optimally.

Hormonal Influences on Carb Utilization

Welcome to the intricate dance of hormones – the conductors of our body's orchestra. In the realm of carb cycling for women over 50, understanding hormonal influences on carb utilization is like mastering the steps to a well-choreographed ballet.

Estrogen and Insulin Sensitivity: As women enter menopause, estrogen levels decline. This hormonal shift can impact insulin sensitivity, affecting how the body responds to carbohydrates. Insulin is the hormone responsible for ushering glucose into cells for energy. A decrease in estrogen can lead to reduced insulin sensitivity, potentially contributing to weight gain and metabolic challenges. Carb cycling offers a strategic approach to managing carbohydrate intake, optimizing insulin sensitivity, and promoting better blood sugar control.

Cortisol and Stress Response: Life's demands can often translate into elevated stress levels, triggering the release of cortisol – the stress hormone. Cortisol can influence carb utilization by promoting the storage of fat, especially around the abdominal area. Carb cycling, with its focus on nutrient timing and strategic carbohydrate manipulation, becomes a valuable tool in modulating cortisol levels and mitigating the impact of stress on metabolic health.

Thyroid Function: The thyroid gland, a key player in metabolism regulation, can also undergo changes with age. Thyroid hormones influence the body's metabolic rate, and imbalances can lead to weight fluctuations. Carb cycling, when tailored to individual hormonal profiles, can help support thyroid function, ensuring that the body's metabolic thermostat remains finely tuned.

Understanding the intricate interplay between hormones and carbohydrate utilization is not about controlling nature but rather about harmonizing with it. Carb cycling emerges as a flexible and personalized strategy that adapts to hormonal nuances, allowing women over 50 to navigate this intricate dance with grace and resilience.

Impact of Carb Cycling on Metabolism

So, how does carb cycling-shake things up in the metabolic arena? Let's explore the profound impact this dietary strategy can have on metabolism, especially for women over 50.

Metabolic Flexibility: One of the key benefits of carb cycling is the promotion of metabolic flexibility. The body becomes adept at efficiently switching between burning carbohydrates and fats for fuel. This flexibility is particularly valuable for women over 50, as it aligns with the body's changing ability to utilize different fuel sources. By incorporating low-carb days strategically, carb cycling encourages the body to tap into stored fat for energy, supporting weight management goals.

Caloric Manipulation: Carb cycling involves varying carbohydrate intake throughout the week, creating a caloric deficit on some days and a surplus on others. This manipulation keeps the metabolism dynamic and prevents it from settling into a stagnant state. For women over 50, whose metabolism may be experiencing a natural decline, this fluctuation can be a gamechanger in maintaining a healthy weight and sustaining energy levels.

Preserving Lean Muscle Mass: As mentioned earlier, muscle mass plays a crucial role in metabolism. Carb cycling, when combined with adequate protein intake and resistance training, becomes a powerful ally in preserving lean muscle mass. This is especially pertinent for women over
50, who may be facing the dual challenge of age-related muscle loss and metabolic cha

CHAPTER 3: GETTING STARTED WITH CARB CYCLING

Assessing Current Dietary Habits

Embarking on the carb cycling journey requires a thoughtful examination of where you currently stand in terms of your dietary habits. It's not about judgment or guilt; it's about gaining clarity on your starting point so you can map out a realistic and sustainable path forward.

Food Journaling: Begin by keeping a detailed food journal for at least a week. Note down everything you eat and drink, including portion sizes and meal timings. This provides a snapshot of your current eating patterns, revealing both strengths and areas that might need adjustment. It's an eye-opening exercise that lays the groundwork for informed decision making.

Nutrient Breakdown: Take a closer look at the macronutrient composition of your meals. How much of your daily intake comes from carbohydrates, proteins, and fats? Understanding this breakdown provides insights into your current nutritional balance. It sets the stage for making targeted adjustments during the carb cycling process, ensuring that your body receives the right proportions of each macronutrient.

Identifying Trigger Foods: Pay attention to foods that might be your Achilles' heel the ones you reach for in moments of stress or comfort. Identifying these trigger foods helps you become aware of potential pitfalls and areas where carb cycling strategies can be particularly beneficial. It's not about deprivation but about making conscious choices that align with your goals.

Meal Timing and Frequency: Consider your meal timing and frequency. Do you tend to skip meals, leading to energy crashes? Or are you a frequent snacker? Understanding your meal patterns helps in structuring an effective carb cycling plan that works seamlessly with your lifestyle.

Emotional and Social Connections: Food is not just fuel; it often carries emotional and social weight. Assess how emotions and social situations impact your-eating habits. This awareness sets the stage for a carb cycling approach that not only supports your physical goals but also nurtures a healthy relationship with food.

The process of assessing your current dietary habits is not a punitive exercise but a compassionate and empowering one. It's about understanding yourself and your relationship with food, creating a solid foundation for the personalized carb cycling journey ahead.

Setting Personalized Goals

With a clear understanding of where you currently stand, the next step in your carb cycling adventure is to define your destination. What are your goals, both short-term and long-term? Personalization is the key here – one size does not fit all, and your goals should reflect your unique aspirations and circumstances.

Clarifying Objectives: Start by clarifying why you're venturing into carb cycling. Is it for weight management, improved energy levels, or optimizing athletic performance? Your objectives act as the guiding stars, shaping the strategies you'll employ and the adjustments you'll make along the way.

Realistic and Achievable Targets: Set realistic and achievable targets that align with your overarching objectives. These targets could be related to weight loss, muscle gain, or specific health markers. Avoid falling into the trap of setting unrealistic goals that could lead to frustration. Instead, celebrate incremental progress and use it as motivation to keep moving forward.

Considering Timeframes: Carb cycling can be approached in various cycles – daily, weekly, or even monthly. Define the timeframe that suits your lifestyle and preferences. Some individuals may prefer a more structured daily approach, while others might find success in weekly or monthly cycles. The key is to find a rhythm that you can sustain over the long haul.

Incorporating Non-Scale Victories: While the scale is a tangible measure of progress, don't forget to incorporate non-scale victories into your goal-setting. These could include improvements in energy levels, enhanced mood, better sleep, or increased strength. These victories provide a holistic perspective on your well-being and contribute to a positive mindset.

Accounting for Individual Factors: Consider individual factors that might influence your goals. Are there any underlying health conditions or medications that need to be taken into account? How does your daily schedule and lifestyle impact your ability to adhere to specific carb cycling strategies?

Tailoring your goals to accommodate these factors ensures a realistic and sustainable approach. Setting personalized goals is about creating a roadmap that resonates with your aspirations and honors your individuality. It's not a one-size-fits-all approach; it's your unique journey, and the goals you set pave the way for a fulfilling and purpose-driven carb cycling experience.

Choosing the Right Carb Cycling Approach

With a clear vision of your starting point and destination, the next crucial step is selecting the right carb cycling approach that aligns with your goals, preferences, and lifestyle. Carb cycling is not a one-dimensional concept; it offers flexibility, allowing you to tailor the approach to suit your unique needs.

Daily Carb Cycling: This approach involves cycling your daily carbohydrate intake, typically alternating between higher and lower carb days. On higher carb days, you might consume more carbohydrates to support intense workouts or higher energy demands, while lower carb days are designed to promote fat burning. This method is well-suited for those who prefer a structured and daily routine.

Weekly Carb Cycling: If the daily ebb and flow seem too intricate, weekly carb cycling might be the perfect fit. This approach involves varying your carb intake on a weekly basis, providing more flexibility. For instance, you might have a few consecutive higher carb days followed by lower carb days. This approach accommodates variations in your weekly schedule and is often favored for its simplicity.

Targeted Carb Cycling: This approach hones in on specific times, such as around workouts. On days when you engage in more demanding physical activity, you strategically increase your carb intake to fuel your workouts and support recovery. This targeted approach is excellent for individuals with specific fitness goals and allows for a more nuanced adjustment of carb intake.

Cyclical Carb Cycling: For those who appreciate a more extended view, cyclical carb cycling involves cycling carbohydrates on a monthly basis. This approach is often used in sync with the menstrual cycle for women, recognizing the hormonal shifts that occur. It provides a broader perspective on carb cycling, accommodating longer-term fluctuations in energy needs and goals.

Experimentation and Adaptation: The beauty of carb cycling lies in its adaptability. It's not a rigid set of rules but a framework that you can adjust based on your responses and preferences. It might take some experimentation to find the sweet spot that works for you. Pay attention to how your body responds, be open to adjustments, and embrace the flexibility that carb cycling offers. Choosing the right carb cycling approach is about finding harmony between your goals, lifestyle, and preferences. It's not a decision set in stone; it's a dynamic choice that evolves as you progress on your carb cycling journey. Remember, the most effective approach is the one that aligns seamlessly with your life and empowers you to achieve your goals with joy and sustainability.

CHAPTER 4: CREATING A CARB CYCLING PLAN

Designing a Weekly Cycle

Creating an effective carb cycling plan involves designing a weekly cycle that harmonizes with your lifestyle, preferences, and fitness goals. The beauty of carb cycling lies in its flexibility, and crafting a weekly cycle allows you to synchronize your nutritional approach with your weekly activities and energy requirements.

High Carb Days: Begin by strategically placing high carb days within your week. These days are designed to coincide with your most demanding physical activities or workout sessions. High carb intake on these days provides the energy needed for optimal performance and recovery. Consider aligning high carb days with strength training or more intense cardio sessions.

Moderate Carb Days: Intersperse moderate carb days throughout the week. These days maintain a balanced carbohydrate intake, providing sustained energy without the higher levels associated with intense workouts. Moderate carb days are like the steady heartbeat of your weekly cycle, ensuring a consistent supply of energy for your body's needs.

Low Carb Days: Allocate a couple of days for low carb intake. These days are characterized by a reduction in overall carbohydrate consumption, promoting the body's reliance on stored fat for energy. Low carb days are valuable for encouraging fat loss, enhancing metabolic flexibility, and supporting overall body composition goals.

Rest or Active Recovery Days: On rest days or active recovery days, your carb intake can be adjusted accordingly. Since the energy demands are lower, you might choose to reduce carbs slightly on these days while maintaining an adequate intake of protein and healthy fats. This adjustment ensures that your nutritional plan aligns with your body's varying energy requirements throughout the week.

Designing a weekly cycle requires a thoughtful consideration of your schedule, workout routine, and personal preferences. It's not a one-size-fits-all approach; it's about tailoring the plan to suit your unique needs and ensuring that your carb cycling journey seamlessly integrates into your life.

Adjusting Carb Intake Based on Activity Levels

The dynamic nature of carb cycling comes to life when you learn to adjust your carbohydrate intake based on your activity levels. Your body's need for carbohydrates fluctuates with the intensity and duration of your workouts, and fine-tuning your carb intake accordingly ensures optimal performance and recovery.

Pre-Workout Nutrition: Fueling your body adequately before a workout is essential for sustained energy and performance. On days with more intense or prolonged exercise, consider increasing your carb intake in the pre-workout meal. Opt for easily digestible carbohydrates, such as fruits or whole grains, to provide a readily available source of energy.

Intra-Workout Nutrition: For extended workouts or activities, especially those lasting more than an hour, incorporating intra-workout nutrition can be beneficial. This might include a sports drink, energy gels, or a carb-rich snack to maintain blood sugar levels and stave off fatigue. Adjusting carb intake during the activity ensures that your body has a continuous supply of energy.

Post-Workout Nutrition: After a workout, your body is in a prime state to replenish glycogen stores and kickstart the recovery process. This is a crucial time to prioritize carbohydrates, especially higher glycemic options, paired with a source of protein. The combination of carbs and protein aids in muscle recovery and replenishes energy stores for your next session.

Rest Days: On days when you're taking a break from intense exercise, your overall energy expenditure is lower. Adjust your carb intake accordingly by slightly reducing the amount of carbohydrates in your meals. This nuanced adjustment ensures that your nutritional plan aligns with your body's varying energy needs, promoting balance and preventing unnecessary calorie surplus.

Understanding how to adjust carb intake based on activity levels is about cultivating a responsive and intuitive approach to nutrition. It's not a rigid formula but a dynamic process that empowers you to finetune your carb cycling plan to support your body's unique d

While carb cycling places a significant emphasis on managing carbohydrate intake, it's crucial to recognize the equally important roles of protein and fat in creating a well-rounded and balanced nutrition plan. These macronutrients play diverse roles in supporting overall health, muscle maintenance, and

sustained energy levels.

Protein's Crucial Role: Protein is the building block of tissues, muscles, enzymes, and hormones. Its importance in a carb cycling plan cannot be overstated. Adequate protein intake supports muscle maintenance, aids in recovery after workouts, and promotes a feeling of fullness, which can be particularly beneficial during lower carb days. Include lean sources of protein such as poultry, fish, tofu, and legumes in each meal to ensure a balanced nutrient profile.

Balancing Healthy Fats: Incorporating healthy fats is essential for several reasons. Fats are a concentrated source of energy, crucial for activities that demand a slower, more sustained release of fuel. They also play a role in hormone production and absorption of fat-soluble vitamins. Include sources of healthy fats such as avocados, nuts, seeds, and olive oil in your meals, ensuring a well-rounded and satisfying nutritional profile.

Timing Matters: Distribute your protein and fat intake strategically throughout the day. Including protein in each meal helps maintain a consistent amino acid pool in the bloodstream, supporting muscle protein synthesis. Similarly, spreading out healthy fats ensures a steady supply of energy and supports overall metabolic health.

Hydration and Micronutrients: Don't forget about hydration and micronutrients. Staying adequately hydrated is crucial for overall well-being and can impact your energy levels. Additionally, ensure that your meals are rich in a variety of colorful fruits and vegetables to provide essential vitamins and minerals.

These micronutrients contribute to your body's overall health and vitality.

Incorporating protein and healthy fats into your carb cycling plan is about achieving balance and comprehensive nourishment. It's a holistic approach that recognizes the importance of each macronutrient in promoting optimal health, performance, and resilience throughout your carb cycling journey.

CHAPTER 5: SAMPLE CARB CYCLING

Daily Meal Plans for Different Carb Cycling Phases

Creating effective and enjoyable meal plans is at the heart of a successful carb cycling journey. Tailoring your daily meals to different carb cycling phases ensures that you meet your energy needs, support your fitness goals, and enjoy a variety of delicious and nourishing foods.

Cooking Tips for Balanced Nutrition

Making carb cycling meals both delicious and nutritious is an art that involves creativity in the kitchen and an understanding of the nutritional components that fuel your body. Here are some recipes and cooking tips to inspire balanced and flavorful meals throughout your carb cycling journey.

1. **Quality Ingredients:**

Start with high-quality, nutrient-dense ingredients. Opt for whole grains, lean proteins, healthy fats, and a variety of fruits and vegetables. Prioritizing fresh, unprocessed foods ensures that you're getting the most nutritional value from your meals.

2   **Balance Macronutrients:**

Aim for a balanced distribution of macronutrients in each meal, regardless of whether it's a high, moderate, or low carb day. Incorporate lean proteins, complex carbohydrates, and healthy fats to support overall health and satiety.

- **Portion Control:**

Practice portion control to prevent overeating and ensure you're consuming the appropriate amount of calories for your individual needs. Use measuring tools to portion out ingredients accurately and avoid mindless eating.

- **Variety and Diversity:**

Embrace variety in your meals by incorporating a diverse range of foods. Experiment with different grains, proteins, and vegetables to keep meals interesting and maximize nutrient intake.

1. **Cooking Methods:**

Choose cooking methods that preserve the nutritional integrity of ingredients. Opt for grilling, baking, steaming, or sautéing over frying to minimize added fats and calories.

2. **Healthy Fats:**
Include sources of healthy fats such as avocados, nuts, seeds, and olive oil in your meals.

These-fat are essential for hormone production, brain health, and nutrient absorption.

3. **Hydration:**

Stay hydrated throughout the day by drinking plenty of water. Hydration is essential for overall health and can help support digestion, metabolism, and energy levels.

4. **Meal Planning and Preparation:**

Plan your meals in advance to ensure that they are balanced and nutritious. Prep ingredients ahead of time to streamline the cooking process and make healthy eating more convenient.

5. **Read Labels:**

Be mindful of food labels and ingredients lists when purchasing packaged foods. Look for products with minimal added sugars, sodium, and unhealthy fats, and prioritize whole food options whenever possible.

6. **Listen to Your Body:**

Pay attention to how different foods make you feel and adjust your carb cycling plan accordingly. Listen to hunger and fullness cues, and honor your body's needs with nourishing, balanced meals.

Portion Control and Mindful Eating

Regardless of the carb cycling phase, practicing portion control and mindful eating is crucial. Use smaller plates to help control portion sizes, and take the time to savor each bite. Pay attention to hunger and fullness cues, and avoid distractions like television or phones.　while eating. This mindful approach enhances the overall dining experience and encourages a healthy relationship with food.

Experimenting with recipes and incorporating cooking tips can transform your carb cycling meals into a culinary adventure. Enjoy the process of discovering new flavors, textures, and combinations that not only align with your nutritional goals but also make each meal a delightful experience.

CHAPTER 6: RECIPES FOR HIGH CARB DAYS

Breakfast

Kickstart your day with a hearty breakfast that includes complex carbohydrates for sustained energy. Try a bowl of oatmeal topped with fresh berries, a sprinkle of nuts, and a dollop of Greek yogurt. This combination provides a mix of fiber, vitamins, and proteins.

1.Banana Nut Pancakes
Prep Time: 10minutes
Cooking Time: 15minutes
Serving Size: 2pancakes
Ingredients:

- 1cup pancake mix
- 1 ripe banana, mashed
- 1/4 cup chopped nuts (walnuts or almonds)
- 1 cup milk
- 1 egg
- 1 tablespoon oil
- Maple syrup for serving

Instructions:

1. In a bowl, mix pancake mix, mashed banana, chopped nuts, milk, egg, and oil until well combined.
2. Heat a griddle or non-stick skillet over medium heat.
3. Pour 1/4 cup of batter for each pancake onto the griddle.
4. Cook until bubbles form on the surface, then flip and cook until golden brown.
5. Serve with maple syrup.

Nutritional Information (Per Serving):

- Calories: 350
- Protein: 8g
- Carbohydrates: 45g
- Fiber: 3g
- Sugars: 12g
- Fat: 15g
- Sodium: 450mg
- Potassium: 250mg

2.Classic French Toast
Prep Time: 10minutes
Cooking Time:10minutes
Serving Size: 2 slices

Ingredients:

- slices of whole-grain bread
- eggs
- 1/2 cup milk
- 1 teaspoon vanilla extract
- 1/2 teaspoon cinnamon
- Butter for cooking
- Fresh berries for topping

Instructions:

1. In a shallow bowl, whisk together eggs, milk, vanilla extract, and cinnamon.
2. Dip each slice of bread into the egg mixture, ensuring it's well-coated In a skillet, melt butter over medium heat.
3. Cook each slice until golden brown on both sides.
4. In a skillet, melt butter over medium heat.
5. Cook each slice until golden brown on both sides.
6. Top with fresh berries and a sprinkle of powdered sugar if desired.

Nutritional Information (Per Serving):

- Calories: 280
- Protein: 12g
- Carbohydrates: 35g
- Fiber: 5g
- Sugars: 8g
- Fat: 10g
- Sodium: 350mg
- Potassium: 180mg

3.Blueberry Oatmeal
Prep Time: 5minutes
Cooking Time: 10minutes
Serving Size: 1 bowl
Ingredients:

- 1/2 cup old-fashioned   oats
- 1 cup milk (or water) 1/2 cup fresh blueberries
- 1 tablespoon honey
- 1 tablespoon chopped nuts (optional)

Instructions:

1. In a saucepan, bring oats and milk to a simmer, stirring occasionally.
2. Cook until oats are tender and the mixture thickens.
3. Stir in blueberries and cook for an additional 2-3 minutes.
4. Drizzle with honey and sprinkle with nuts.
5. Serve warm.

Nutritional Information (Per Serving):

- Calories: 300
- Protein: 9g
- Carbohydrates: 50g
- Fiber: 7g
- Sugars: 18g
- Fat: 6g
- Sodium: 80mg
- Potassium: 280mg

4.High-Protein Yogurt Parfait
Prep Time: 5minutes
CookinTime: 5minutes
Serving Size: 1 parfait
Ingredients:

- cup Greek yogurt
- 1/2 cup granola
- 1/2 cup mixed berries
- 1 tablespoon honey

Instructions:

1. In a glass, layer Greek yogurt, granola, and mixed berries.
2. Repeat the layers as desired.
3. Drizzle with honey.
4. Serve immediately.

Nutritional Information (Per Serving):

- Calories: 350
- Protein: 20g
- Carbohydrates: 45g
- Fiber: 6g
- Sugars: 15g

- Fat: 10g
- Sodium: 120mg
- Potassium: 320mg

5.Chocolate and banana Smoothie
Prep Time:5minutes
Cooking Time:5minutes
Serving: 1 bowl
Ingredients:

- 1 frozen banana
- cup milk (or almond milk)
- 2tablespoons cocoa powder
- tablespoon peanut butter
- Toppings: sliced banana, chia seeds, shredded coconut

Instructions:

1. In a blender, combine frozen banana, milk, cocoa powder, and peanut butter.
2. Blend until smooth and creamy.
3. Pour into a bowl and top with sliced banana, chia seeds, and shredded coconut.
4. Enjoy with a spoon.

Nutritional Information (Per Serving):

- Calories: 400
- Protein: 15g
- Carbohydrates: 60g
- Fiber: 9g
- Sugars: 30g
- Fat: 14g
- Sodium: 150mg
- Potassium: 450mg

6.Vegetable and Cheese
Prep Time:10minutes
Cooking Time:10minutes
Serving :1 omelette
Ingredients:

- eggs
- 1/4 cup diced bell peppers
- 1/4 cup diced tomatoes
- 1/4 cup shredded cheese
- Salt and pepper to taste
- Fresh herbs for garnish

Instructions:

1. In a bowl, whisk eggs and season with salt and pepper.
2. Heat a non-stick skillet over medium heat.
3. Pour eggs into the skillet and let them set for a moment.

4. Sprinkle bell peppers, tomatoes, and cheese over one half of the omelette.
5. Fold the other half over the filling.
6. Cook until the cheese melts and the eggs are cooked through.
7. Garnish with fresh herbs.

Nutritional Information (Per Serving):

- Calories: 320
- Protein: 18g
- Carbohydrates: 5g
- Fiber: 1g
- Sugars: 2g
- Fat: 25g
- Sodium: 350mg
- Potassium: 280mg

7.Peanut Butter Banana Toast

Prep Time: 5minutes

CookinTime:5minutes

ServingSize:2slices

Ingredients:

- slices whole-grain bread
- 2 tablespoons peanut butter
- 1 banana, sliced
- Drizzle of honey (optional)

Instructions:

1. Toast the slices of bread to your liking.
2. Spread peanut butter evenly on each slice.
3. Arrange banana slices on top.
4.   Drizzle with honey if desired.
5. Serve immediately.

Nutritional Information (Per Serving):

- Calories: 320
- Protein: 10g
- Carbohydrates: 45g
- Fiber: 6g
- Sugars: 15g
- Fat: 12g
- Sodium: 250mg
- Potassium: 300mg

Lunch

Opt for a balanced lunch that includes a lean protein source, whole grains, and plenty of colorful vegetables. Grilled chicken or tofu paired with quinoa or brown rice and a generous portion of mixed vegetables creates a satisfying and nutritionally rich meal.

1.Sweet Potato and Black Bean Burrito Bowl
Prep Time: 20minutes
Cooking Time: 30minutes
Serving Size: 2
Ingredients:

- 1 cup brown rice, cooked
- 1 sweet potato, cubed
- 1 can black beans, drained and rinsed
- 1 cup corn kernels (fresh or frozen)
- 1 avocado, sliced
- 1/2 cup salsa
- 1/4 cup Greek yogurt
- Fresh cilantro for garnish

Instructions:

1. Roast sweet potato cubes in the oven until tender.
2. in a bowl, assemble cooked brown rice, roasted sweet potatoes, black beans, corn, and avocado slices
3. Top with salsa, Greek yogurt, and garnish with fresh cilantro.
4. Mix well before serving.

Nutritional Information (Per Serving):

- Calories: 480
- Protein: 14g
- Carbohydrates: 80g
- Fiber: 15g
- Sugars: 6g
- Fat: 15g
- Sodium: 450mg
- Potassium: 700mg

2.Mediterranean Quinoa Bowl

Prep Time: 15minutes
Cooking Time: 15minutes
Serving Size: 2

Ingredients:
- 1 cup quinoa, cooked
- 1 cup cherry tomatoes, halved
- 1/2 cucumber, diced
- 1/4 cup Kalamata olives, sliced
- 1/4 cup red onion, finely chopped
- 1/2 cup feta cheese, crumbled
- 2 tablespoons olive oil
- 1 tablespoon red wine vinegar
- 1 teaspoon dried oregano
- Salt and pepper to taste

Instructions:
1. In a bowl, combine cooked quinoa, cherry tomatoes, cucumber, olives, red onion, and feta cheese.
2. In a small bowl, whisk together olive oil, red wine vinegar, dried oregano, salt, and pepper
3. Drizzle the dressing over the quinoa mixture and toss gently.
4. Serve at room temperature.

Nutritional Information (Per Serving):
- Calories: 420
- Protein: 12g
- Carbohydrates: 55g
- Fiber: 8g
- Sugars: 4g
- Fat: 18g
- Sodium: 550mg
- Potassium: 500mg

3.Mango Avocado Quinoa Salad
PrepTime: 15minutes
CookingTime: 15minutes
Serving Size: 2
Ingredients:
- 1 cup quinoa, cooked
- 1 mango, diced
- 1 avocado, diced
- 1/2 red onion, finely chopped
- 1/4 cup fresh cilantro, chopped
- Juice of 1 lime
- 2 tablespoons olive oil
- Salt and pepper to taste

Instructions:

1. In a large bowl, combine cooked quinoa, diced mango, avocado, chopped red onion, and cilantro.
2. In a small bowl, whisk together lime juice, olive oil, salt, and pepper.
3. Pour the dressing over the salad and toss gently.
4. Serve chilled.

Nutritional Information (Per Serving):

- Calories: 420
- Protein: 10g
- Carbohydrates: 65g
- Fiber: 10g
- Sugars: 8g
- Fat: 15g
- Sodium: 350mg
- Potassium: 700mg

4.Lentil and Vegetable Stir-Fry

Prep Time:20minutes
Cooking Time:15minutes
Serving Size:2
Ingredients:

- cup lentils, cooked
- cup broccoli florets
- 1 bell pepper, sliced
- 1carrot, julienned
- 1cup snap peas   3 tablespoons soy sauce
- 1 tablespoon sesame oil
- 1 teaspoon ginger, minced
- 2 cloves garlic, minced

Instructions:

1. In a wok or large skillet, heat sesame oil over medium-high heat.
2. Add ginger and garlic, stir-fry for 30 seconds.
3. Add broccoli, bell pepper, carrot, and snap peas. Stir-fry until vegetables are tender-crisp.
4. Add cooked lentils and soy sauce. Toss until well combined.
5. Serve hot.

Nutritional Information (Per Serving):

- Calories: 420
- Protein: 20g
- Carbohydrates: 60g
- Fiber: 15g
- Sugars: 6g
- Fat: 10g
- Sodium: 700mg

- Potassium: 800mg

5.Pasta Primavera with Roasted Vegetables
Prep Time:20 minutes
Cooking Time:20 minutes
Serving Size: 2
Ingredients:

- cups whole-grain pasta, cooked
- 1 zucchini, sliced
- 1 yellow squash, sliced
- 1 cup cherry tomatoes, halved
- 1 bell pepper, sliced
- 1/4 cup Parmesan cheese, grated
- 2 tablespoons olive oil
- 2 cloves garlic, minced
- 1 teaspoon Italian seasoning
- Salt and pepper to taste

Instructions:

1. Preheat the oven to 400°F (200°C).
2. Toss zucchini, yellow squash, cherry tomatoes, and bell pepper with olive oil, minced garlic, Italian seasoning, salt, and pepper.
3. Roast in the oven until vegetables are tender.
4. Cook pasta according to package instructions.
5. Mix roasted vegetables with cooked pasta and top with grated Parmesan cheese.
6. Serve warm.

Nutritional Information (Per Serving):

- Calories: 480g
- Protein: 15g
- Carbohydrates: 75g
- Fiber: 12g
- Sugars: 6g
- Fat: 15g
- Sodium: 350g
- Potassium: 700mg

6.Tomato Basil Quinoa Risotto
Prep Time:10minutes
Cooking Time:25minutes
Serving Size:2
Ingredients:

- 1cup quinoa, rinsed
- 1cups vegetable broth
- 2onion, finely chopped
- 1cloves garlic, minced

- 1up cherry tomatoes, halved
- 1/4 cup fresh basil, chopped
- 1/4 cup Parmesan cheese, grated
- 1tablespoons olive oil
- Salt and pepper to taste

Instructions:

1. In a saucepan, sauté chopped onion and garlic in olive oil until softened.
2. Add quinoa and cook for 1-2 minutes.
3. Gradually add vegetable broth, one cup at a time, stirring frequently until absorbed.
4. Continue adding broth and stirring until quinoa is cooked.
5. Stir in cherry tomatoes, fresh basil, Parmesan cheese, salt, and pepper.
6. Serve hot.

Nutritional Information (Per Serving):

- Calories: 420
- Protein: 15g
- Carbohydrates: 60g
- Fiber: 8g
- Sugars: 4g
- Fat: 18g
- Sodium: 700mg
- Potassium: 600mg

7.Vegetarian Stuffed Bell Peppers

Prep Time:20minutes
Cooking Time:30minutes
Serving Size: 2
Ingredients:

- bell peppers, halved and seeds removed
- 1 cup quinoa, cooked
- 1 can black beans, drained and rinsed
- 1 cup corn kernels (fresh or frozen)
- 1 cup diced tomatoes
- 1/2 cup shredded cheddar cheese
- 1 tablespoon olive oil
- 1 teaspoon cumin
- 1 teaspoon chili powder
- Salt and pepper to taste

Instructions:

1. Preheat the oven to 375°F (190°C).
2. In a bowl, mix cooked quinoa, black beans, corn, diced tomatoes, olive oil, cumin, chili powder, salt, and pepper.

3. Stuff each bell pepper half with the quinoa mixture.
4. Top with shredded cheddar cheese.
5. Bake in the oven until peppers are tender and cheese is melted.
6. Serve warm.

Nutritional Information (Per Serving):

- Calories: 480
- Protein: 18g
- Carbohydrates: 75g
- Fiber: 15g
- Sugars: 5g
- Fat: 15g
- Sodium: 550mg
- Potassium: 700mg

Snacks

Keep your energy levels up with a mid-afternoon snack. Consider a fruit smoothie with banana, berries, spinach, and a scoop of protein powder. This snack provides a nutrient boost and helps bridge the gap between meals.

1.Apple Slices with Peanut Butter
Prep Time: 5minutes
Cooking Time: NA
Serving Size: 1
Ingredients:
- 1 medium apple, sliced
- 2 tablespoons natural peanut butter

Instructions:
1. Slice the apple into thin wedges.
2. Spread peanut butter on each apple slice.
3. Arrange on a plate and serve.

Nutritional Information (Per Serving):
- Calories: 230
- Protein: 7g
- Carbohydrates: 25g
- Fiber: 5g
- Sugars: 15g
- Fat: 13g
- Sodium: 90mg
- Potassium: 250mg

2.Hummus and Veggie Sticks
Prep Time:10minutes
Cooking Time: NA
Serving Size: 1
Ingredients:
- 1/2 cup hummus
- 1 cup carrot and cucumber sticks

Instructions:
1. Arrange carrot and cucumber sticks on a plate.
2. Serve with hummus for dipping.

Nutritional Information (Per Serving):
- Calories: 180
- Protein: 6g
- Carbohydrates: 20g
- Fiber: 7g
- Sugars: 5g

- Fat: 10g
- Sodium: 300mg
- Potassium: 500mg

3.Banana Berry Smoothie

Prep Time:10minutes
Cooking Time: NA
Serving Size: 1
Ingredients:

- 1 ripe banana
- 1/2 cup mixed berries (strawberries, blueberries, raspberries)
- 1 cup unsweetened almond milk
- 1 tablespoon chia seeds

Instructions:

1. In a blender, combine banana, mixed berries, almond milk, and chia seeds.
2. Blend until smooth.
3. Pour into a glass and enjoy.

Nutritional Information (Per Serving):

- Calories: 220
- Protein: 4g
- Carbohydrates: 40g
- Fiber: 10g
- Sugars: 18g
- Fat: 7g
- Sodium: 120mg
- Potassium: 450mg

4.Rice Cake with Cottage Cheese and Pineapple

Prep Time: 5minutes
CookingTime: N/A
Serving Size:1
Ingredients:

- 1rice cake
- 1/2 cup low-fat cottage cheese
- 1/2 cup fresh pineapple chunks

Instructions:

1. Spread cottage cheese over the rice cake.
2. Top with fresh pineapple chunks.
3. Enjoy this light and tasty snack.

Nutritional Information (Per Serving):

- Calories: 180
- Protein: 10g
- Carbohydrates: 30g
- Fiber: 2g
- Sugars: 14g
- Fat: 3g

- Sodium: 280mg
- Potassium: 220mg

5.Sweet Potato Toast with Avocado

Prep Time:10minutes

Cooking Time: 15 minutes

Serving Size: 1

Ingredients:

- 1sweet potato, sliced
- 1/2 avocado, sliced
- 1 teaspoon olive oil
- Salt and pepper to taste

Instructions:

1. Preheat the oven to 400°F (200°C).
2. Place sweet potato slices on a baking sheet.
3. Drizzle with olive oil, salt, and pepper.
4. Bake until sweet potato is tender.
5. Top with sliced avocado and serve.

Nutritional Information (Per Serving):

- Calories: 220
- Protein: 3g
- Carbohydrates: 30g
- Fiber: 7g
- Sugars: 6g
- Fat: 10g
- Sodium: 10mg
- Potassium: 480mg

6.Whole Grain Crackers with Cheese and Grapes

Prep Time:5minutes

Cooking Time: N/A   **Serving**

Size: 1   **Ingredients:**

- 8-10 whole grain crackers
- 1 ounce cheese (cheddar, gouda, or your choice)
- 1/2 cup red or green grapes

Instructions:

1. Arrange whole grain crackers on a plate.
2. Place slices of cheese on top.
3. Serve with grapes on the side.

Nutritional Information (Per Serving):

- Calories: 280
- Protein: 8g
- Carbohydrates: 30g
- Fiber: 4g

- Sugars: 12g
- Fat: 14g
- Sodium: 220mg
- Potassium: 230mg

7. Peanut Butter and Banana Wrap

Prep Time: 8minute
Cooking Time: NA
Serving Size: 1
Ingredients:

- 1 whole wheat tortilla
- 2 tablespoons natural peanut butter
- 1 banana, sliced

Instructions:

1. Spread peanut butter over the whole wheat tortilla.
2. Place banana slices in the center.
3. Fold the sides and roll it into a wrap.
4. Slice in half and enjoy.

Nutritional Information (Per Serving):

- Calories: 340
- Protein: 8g
- Carbohydrates: 45g
- Fiber: 6g
- Sugars: 16g
- Fat: 16g
- Sodium: 190mg
- Potassium: 450mg

Dinner

Wrap up your high carb day with a well-rounded dinner. Baked salmon with sweet potato wedges and steamed broccoli offers a combination of protein, complex carbohydrates, and essential nutrients. It's a delicious and satisfying way to end your day.

1. Mushroom and Spinach Stuffed Sweet Potatoes

Prep Time: 10minutes

Cooking Time: 45minutes

Serving Size: 2

Ingredients:

- medium sweet potatoes
- 1 tablespoon olive oil
- 1 cup mushrooms, chopped
- 2 cups fresh spinach
- 2 cloves garlic, minced
- Salt and pepper to taste
- 1/4 cup feta cheese, crumbled

Instructions:

1. Preheat the oven to 400°F (200°C).
2. Wash sweet potatoes and prick them with a fork. Bake for 40-45 minutes until tender.
3. In a pan, heat olive oil. Add garlic and sauté until golden.
4. Add mushrooms and cook until softened. Add spinach and cook until wilted.
5. Cut sweet potatoes in half and fluff the insides with a fork.
6. Fill each sweet potato with the mushroom and spinach mixture.
7. Top with crumbled feta.
8. Bake for an additional 5 minutes until cheese melts.
9. Serve hot.

Nutritional Information (Per Serving):

- Calories: 380
- Protein: 8g
- Carbohydrates: 60g
- Fiber: 10g
- Sugars: 12g
- Fat: 12g
- Sodium: 320mg
- Potassium: 900mg

2.Lentil and Brown Rice Casserole

Prep Time:20minute

Cooking Time:40minutes
Serving Size: 4
Ingredients:

- 1 cup brown rice, cooked
  - 1 cup green lentils, cooked
  - 1 tablespoon olive oil
  - 1 onion, diced
  - 2 carrots, diced
  - 2 celery stalks, diced
  - 2 cloves garlic, minced
  - 1 can (14 oz) diced tomatoes
  - 1 teaspoon dried thyme
  - 1 teaspoon paprika
  - 2 cups vegetable broth
  - Salt and pepper to taste
  - 1/4 cup chopped parsley for garnish

Instructions:

1. Preheat the oven to 375°F (190°C).
2. In a large oven-safe pan, heat olive oil over medium heat. Add onions, carrots, celery, and garlic. Sauté until vegetables are softened.
3. Add diced tomatoes, thyme, paprika, salt, and pepper. Stir well.
4. Add cooked brown rice and lentils to the vegetable mixture.
5. Pour vegetable broth over the mixture and stir.
6. Cover the pan with a lid or foil and bake for 30 minutes.
7. Remove the cover and bake for an additional 10 minutes until the top is golden.
8. Garnish with chopped parsley and serve.

Nutritional Information (Per Serving):

- Calories: 380
- Protein: 18g
- Carbohydrates: 65g
- Fiber: 15g
- Sugars: 6g
- Fat: 6g
- Sodium: 600mg
- Potassium: 900mg

3.Pasta Primavera with Roasted Vegetables
Prep Time: 15minutes
Cooking Time:20minutes
Serving Size: 2

Ingredients:

- cups whole wheat pasta, cooked
- 1 tablespoon olive oil
- 1 zucchini, sliced
- 1 yellow squash, sliced
- 1 bell pepper, sliced
- 1 carrot, julienned

- 2 cloves garlic, minced
- 1 teaspoon dried Italian-herbs
- Salt and pepper to taste
- Grated Parmesan cheese for garnish

Instructions:

1. In a large pan, heat olive oil over medium-high heat.
2. Add garlic and sauté until fragrant.
3. Add zucchini, yellow squash, bell pepper, and carrot. Roast until vegetables are tender-crisp.
4. Sprinkle Italian herbs, salt, and pepper over the vegetables. Stir well.
5. Add cooked whole wheat pasta to the pan. Toss until pasta is coated with the vegetable mixture.
6. Garnish with grated Parmesan cheese and serve.

Nutritional Information (Per Serving):

- Calories: 420
- Protein: 12g
- Carbohydrates: 70g
- Fiber: 12g
- Sugars: 8g
- Fat: 10g
- Sodium: 220mg
- Potassium: 750mg

4.Sweet Potato and Black Bean Quesadillas
Prep Time:15minutes
Cooking Time:15minutes
Serving Size: 2
Ingredients:

- whole wheat tortillas
- 1 large sweet potato, cooked and mashed
- 1 can (15 oz) black beans, drained and rinsed
- 1 cup corn kernels
- 1 teaspoon cumin
- 1/2 teaspoon chili powder
- 1 cup shredded cheddar cheese
- Fresh cilantro for garnish
- Greek yogurt for serving

Instructions:

1. In a bowl, mix mashed sweet potato, black beans, corn, cumin, and chili powder.
2. Place a tortilla on a flat surface. Spread a portion of the sweet potato mixture evenly.
3. Sprinkle shredded cheddar cheese over the mixture.
4. Top with another tortilla to make a quesadilla.
5. Repeat for the remaining tortillas.
6. In a non-stick pan, cook each quesadilla for 3-4 minutes on each side until golden and

cheese is melted.

7. Cut into wedges, garnish with fresh cilantro, and serve with Greek yogurt.
8. 1 cup shredded cheddar cheese
9. Fresh cilantro for garnish
10. Greek yogurt for serving

Nutritional Information (Per Serving):

- Calories: 480
- Protein: 16g
- Carbohydrates: 75g
- Fiber: 15g
- Sugars: 6g
- Fat: 15g
- Sodium: 550mg
- Potassium: 850mg

5.Mediterranean Quinoa Salad

Prep Time:20minutes

Cooking Time:15minutes

Serving Size: 2

Ingredients:

- cup quinoa, cooked
- 1 cucumber, diced
- 1cup cherry tomatoes, halved
- 1/2 red onion, finely chopped
- 1/4 cup Kalamata olives, sliced
- 1/4 cup feta cheese, crumbled
- 2 tablespoons olive oil
- 1tablespoon red wine vinegar
- 1 teaspoon dried oregano
- Salt and pepper to taste
- Fresh parsley for garnish

Instructions:

1. In a large bowl, combine quinoa, cucumber, cherry tomatoes, red onion, olives, and feta cheese.
2. In a small bowl, whisk together olive oil, red wine vinegar, dried oregano, salt, and pepper.
3. Pour the dressing over the quinoa mixture and toss to combine.
4. Garnish with fresh parsley and serve.

Nutritional Information (Per Serving):

- Calories: 380
- Protein: 10g
- Carbohydrates: 55g
- Fiber: 8g
- Sugars: 4g

- Fat: 14g
- Sodium: 400mg
- Potassium: 600mg

6.Spinach and Chickpea Stuffed Bell Peppers

Prep Time:20minutes

Cooking Time:25minutes

Serving Size: 2

Ingredients:

- bell peppers, halved and seeds removed
- 1 tablespoon olive oil
- 1 onion, diced
- 2 cloves garlic, minced
- 1 can (15 oz) chickpeas, drained and rinsed
- 2 cups fresh spinach
- 1 teaspoon cumin
- 1/2 teaspoon smoked paprika
- 1 cup cooked quinoa
- Salt and pepper to taste
- Shredded mozzarella cheese for topping

Instructions:

1. Preheat the oven to 375°F (190°C).
2. In a pan, heat olive oil over medium heat. Add onions and garlic. Sauté until onions are translucent.
3. Add chickpeas, spinach, cumin, and smoked paprika. Cook until spinach is wilted and chickpeas are heated through.
4. Remove the pan from heat and stir in cooked quinoa. Season with salt and pepper.
5. Fill each bell pepper half with the chickpea and quinoa mixture.
6. Top with shredded mozzarella cheese.
7. Bake for 20-25 minutes until the peppers are tender and the cheese is melted.
8. Serve hot.

Nutritional Information (Per Serving):

- Calories: 420
- Protein: 16g
- Carbohydrates: 65g
- Fiber: 12g
- Sugars: 8g
- Fat: 12g
- Sodium: 500mg
- Potassium: 850mg

7.CapreseAvocado Toast

Prep Time:10minutes

Cooking Time:5minutes

Serving Size: 2

Ingredients:

- slices whole grain bread, toasted
- 1 large avocado, sliced
- 1 cup cherry tomatoes, halved
- Fresh mozzarella cheese, sliced
- Balsamic glaze for drizzling
- Fresh basil leaves for garnish
- Salt and pepper to taste

Instructions:

1. Toast the slices of whole grain bread until golden.
2. Arrange avocado slices on each piece of toast.
3. Top with halved cherry tomatoes and slices of fresh mozzarella cheese.
4. Drizzle with balsamic glaze.
5. Garnish with fresh basil leaves and season with salt and pepper.
6. Serve immediately.

Nutritional Information (Per Serving):

- Calories: 380
- Protein: 12g
- Carbohydrates: 50g
- Fiber: 10g
- Sugars: 6g
- Fat: 18g
- Sodium: 320mg
- Potassium: 700mg

CHAPTER 7: RECIPES FOR MODERATE CARB DAYS

Breakfast

Start your morning with a protein-packed breakfast to keep you fueled. A spinach and feta omelet with whole-grain toast offers a balance of protein, healthy fats, and moderate carbs.

1.Greek Yogurt Parfait with Berries
Prep Time:10minutes
Cooking Time:0minutes
Serving Size: 1
Ingredients:
- cup Greek yogurt
- 1/2 cup mixed berries (strawberries, blueberries, raspberries)
- 1/4 cup granola
- 1 tablespoon honey
- 1 teaspoon chia seeds (optional)

Instructions:
1. In a glass or bowl, layer Greek yogurt.
2. Add a layer of mixed berries.
3. Sprinkle granola over the berries.
4. Drizzle honey on top.
5. Optionally, sprinkle chia seeds for added nutrition.
6. Repeat the layers as desired.
7. Serve immediately.

Nutritional Information (Per Serving):
- Calories: 300
- Protein: 20g
- Carbohydrates: 40g
- Fiber: 6g
- Sugars: 20g
- Fat: 8g
- Sodium: 80mg
- Potassium: 400mg

2.Avocado and Tomato Breakfast Sandwich
Prep Time:15minutes
Cooking Time:5minutes
Serving Size: 1

Ingredients:
- 1 whole grain English muffin, toasted

- 1/2 avocado, sliced
- 1 medium tomato, sliced
- 1 poached egg
- Salt and pepper to taste
- Fresh herbs for garnish (optional)

Instructions:

1. Toast the whole grain English muffin.
2. Layer avocado slices on the bottom half.
3. Add tomato slices on top of the avocado.
4. Place a poached egg on the tomatoes.
5. Season with salt and pepper.
6. Garnish with fresh herbs if desired.
7. Top with the other half of the English muffin.
8. Serve immediately.

Nutritional Information (Per Serving):

- Calories: 350
- Protein: 15g
- Carbohydrates: 30g
- Fiber: 8g
- Sugars: 2g
- Fat: 20g
- Sodium: 200mg
- Potassium: 500mg

3.Banana Walnut Pancakes

Prep Time: 15minutes

Cooking Time: 15minutes

Serving Size:2

Ingredients:

- cup whole wheat flour
- 1 tablespoon sugar
- 1 teaspoon baking powder
- 1/2 teaspoon baking soda
- 1tablespoons melted butter
- ripe banana, mashed
- 1/4 cup chopped walnuts

Instructions:

1 In a bowl, whisk together flour, sugar, baking powder, baking soda, and salt.
2 In another bowl, mix buttermilk, egg, and melted butter.
3 Add the wet ingredients to the dry ingredients and stir until just combined.
4 Fold in mashed banana and chopped walnuts.
5 Heat a griddle or non-stick pan over medium heat.

6   Pour 1/4 cup of batter onto the griddle for each pancake.

7   Cook until bubbles form on the surface, then flip and cook the other side.

8   Repeat with the remaining batter.

9   Serve warm with your favorite toppings.

Nutritional Information (Per Serving):

- Calories: 400
- Protein: 10g
- Carbohydrates: 60g
- Fiber: 8g
- Sugars: 10g
- Fat: 15g
- Sodium: 500mg
- Potassium: 400mg

4.Spinach and Feta Omelette

Prep Time:10minutes

Cooking Time:5minutes

Serving Size: 1

Ingredients:

- large eggs
- 1 cup fresh spinach, chopped
- 2 tablespoons crumbled feta cheese
- 1/4 cup cherry tomatoes, halved
- Salt and pepper to taste
- 1 teaspoon olive oil

Instructions:

1. In a bowl, beat the eggs with salt and pepper.
2. Heat olive oil in a non-stick skillet over medium heat.
3. Add chopped spinach and cook until wilted.
4. Pour the beaten eggs over the spinach.
5. Sprinkle feta cheese and cherry tomatoes over one half of the omelette.
6. When the edges start to set, fold the other half over the filling.
7. Cook until the eggs are fully set.
8. Slide the omelette onto a plate and serve.

Nutritional Information (Per Serving):

- Calories: 280
- Protein: 18g
- Carbohydrates: 5g
- Fiber: 2g
- Sugars: 2g
- Fat: 20g
- Sodium: 380mg
- Potassium: 400mg

5.Blueberry Almond Smoothie Bowl

Prep Time:10minutes
Cooking Time:0minutes
ServingSize:1
Ingredients:

- 1 cup frozen blueberries
- 1/2 banana
- 1/2 cup almond-milk
- 1 tablespoon almond butter
- Toppings: sliced almonds, chia seeds, fresh blueberries

Instructions:

1. In a blender, combine frozen blueberries, banana, almond milk, and almond butter.
2. Blend until smooth.
3. Pour the smoothie into a bowl.
4. Top with sliced almonds, chia seeds, and fresh blueberries.
5. Serve immediately.

Nutritional Information (Per Serving):

- Calories: 320
- Protein: 8g
- Carbohydrates: 40g
- Fiber: 10g
- Sugars: 20g
- Fat: 15g
- Sodium: 180mg
- Potassium: 450mg

6.Quinoa Breakfast Bowl

Prep Time:15minutes
Cooking Time:15minutes
Serving Size: 1
Ingredients:

- 1/2 cup cooked quinoa
- 1/2 cup plain Greek yogurt
- 1/2 cup mixed berries (strawberries, blueberries, raspberries) tablespoon honey
- 1tablespoon chopped nuts (almonds, walnuts)

Instructions:

1. In a bowl, layer cooked quinoa.
2. Add a layer of plain Greek yogurt.
3. Top with mixed berries.
4. Drizzle honey over the berries.
5. Sprinkle chopped nuts on top.

6. Serve and enjoy.

Nutritional Information (Per Serving):

- Calories: 300
- Protein: 15g
- Carbohydrates: 40g
- Fiber: 6g
- Sugars: 20g
- Fat: 10g
- Sodium: 80mg
- Potassium: 350mg

7.Whole Wheat Banana Pancakes

Prep Time:15minutes

Cooking Time:15minutes

ServingSize:2

Ingredients:

- cup whole wheat flour
- tablespoon sugar
- 1teaspoonbaking powder
- 1/2teaspoonbaking soda
- 1/4 teaspoon salt
- 1 cup buttermilk
- 1 large egg
- 2tablespoons melted butter
- 1 ripe banana, mashed

Instructions:

1. In a bowl, whisk together whole wheat flour, sugar, baking powder, baking soda, and salt.
2. In another bowl, mix buttermilk, egg, and melted butter.
3. Add the wet ingredients to the dry ingredients and stir until just combined.
4. Fold in mashed banana.
5. Heat a griddle or non-stick pan over medium heat.
6. Pour 1/4 cup of batter onto the griddle for each pancake.
7. Cook until bubbles form on the surface, then flip and cook the other side.
8. Repeat with the remaining batter.
9. Serve warm with your favorite toppings.

Nutritional Information (Per Serving):

- Calories: 350
- Protein: 12g
- Carbohydrates: 50g

- Fiber: 8g
- Sugars: 10g
- Fat: 12g
- Sodium: 500mg
- Potassium: 400mg

Lunch

For lunch, opt for a grilled vegetable and chickpea salad. Load up on nutrient-dense vegetables, legumes for added protein, and a light vinaigrette dressing. It's a refreshing and satisfying choice for a moderate carb day.

1.Salmon and Quinoa Bowl
Prep Time:15minutes
CookingTime:15minutes
ServingSize:1
Ingredients:

- 1/2 cup quinoa, cooked
- ½ 2pound salmon fillet
- 1 tablespoon olive oil
- 1 teaspoon lemon zest
- 1 clove garlic, minced
- Salt and pepper to taste
- 1 cup broccoli florets, steamed
- 1/2 avocado, sliced
- 1 tablespoon soy sauce (low sodium)

Instructions:

1. Season the salmon fillet with olive oil, lemon zest, minced garlic, salt, and pepper.
2. Grill or bake the salmon until flaky.
3. In a bowl, assemble the quinoa, steamed broccoli, and sliced avocado.
4. Place the grilled salmon on top.
5. Drizzle with soy sauce.
6. Serve immediately.

Nutritional Information (Per Serving):

- Calories: 500
- Protein: 30g
- Carbohydrates: 30g
- Fiber: 8g
- Sugars: 2g
- Fat: 30g
- Sodium: 600mg
- Potassium:800mg

2.Turkey and Avocado Wrap
Prep Time:15minutes
Cooking Time:0minutes
Serving Size: 1
Ingredients:

- 1 whole wheat wrap
  - oz turkey breast slices
  - 1/2 avocado, sliced
  - 1/4 cup shredded lettuce
  - 1 tablespoon Greek yogurt
  - 1 teaspoon Dijon mustard
  - Salt and pepper to taste

Instructions:
1. Lay the whole wheat wrap flat on a clean surface.
2. Spread Greek yogurt and Dijon mustard evenly over the wrap.
3. Layer turkey breast slices, avocado slices, and shredded lettuce.
4. Season with salt and pepper to taste.
5. Roll the wrap tightly.
6. Slice in half and serve.

Nutritional Information (Per Serving):
- Calories: 370
- Protein: 30g
- Carbohydrates: 30g
- Fiber: 8g
- Sugars: 2g
- Fat: 18g
- Sodium: 600mg
- Potassium: 500mg

3.Chicken and Vegetable Brown Rice Bowl
Prep Time: 2 minutes
Cooking Time:25minutes
Serving Size: 1
Ingredients:

- 1/2 cup brown rice, cooked
- 4 oz grilled chicken breast, sliced
- 1 cup mixed vegetables (carrots, broccoli, bell peppers)
- 1 tablespoon olive oil
- 1 tablespoon soy sauce (low sodium)
- 1 clove garlic, minced
- Sesame seeds for garnish

Instructions:

1. In a skillet, heat olive oil over medium-high heat.
2. Add minced garlic and sauté for 30 seconds.
3. Add mixed vegetables and cook until tender-crisp.
4. Add sliced grilled chicken to the skillet.
5. Pour soy sauce over the mixture and toss to combine.
6. In a bowl, assemble cooked brown rice.
7. Top with the chicken and vegetable stir-fry.
8. Garnish with sesame seeds.
9. Serve hot.

Nutritional Information (Per Serving):

- Calories: 480
- Protein: 28g
- Carbohydrates: 50g
- Fiber: 8g
- Sugars: 4g
- Fat: 20g
- Sodium: 550mg
- Potassium: 700mg

4.Shrimp and Quinoa Salad

Prep Time:15minutes
Cooking Time:15minutes
Serving Size: 1
Ingredients:

- 1/2 cup quinoa, cooked
- 6 large shrimp, peeled and deveined
- 1 tablespoon olive oil
- 1 teaspoon smoked paprika
- 1/2 teaspoon cumin
- 1/4 teaspoon cayenne pepper
- 1 cup mixed salad greens
- 1/2 cup cherry tomatoes, halved 1/4 cup cucumber, diced
- 1 tablespoon feta cheese, crumbled
- 1 tablespoon balsamic vinaigrette

Instructions:

1. Season shrimp with smoked paprika, cumin, and cayenne pepper.
2. In a skillet, heat olive oil over medium-high heat.
3. Cook shrimp until opaque, about 2-3 minutes per side.
4. In a bowl, combine quinoa, salad greens, cherry tomatoes, cucumber, and feta cheese.
5. Place the cooked shrimp on top.
6. Drizzle with balsamic vinaigrette.
7. Serve chilled.

Nutritional Information (Per Serving):

- Calories: 420

- Protein: 28g
- Carbohydrates: 35g
- Fiber: 6g
- Sugars: 4g
- Fat: 18g
- Sodium: 580mg
- Potassium: 600mg

5.Black Bean and Corn Salad
Prep Time:15minutes
Cooking Time:10minutes
Serving Size: 2
Ingredients:

- 1 can (15 oz) black beans, drained and rinsed

- 1 cup corn kernels (fresh or frozen)

- 1/2 red bell pepper, diced

- 1/4 cup red onion, finely chopped

- 1/4 cup cilantro, chopped

- Juice of 1 lime

- 1 tablespoon olive oil   Salt and pepper to taste

- Avocado slices for garnish

Instructions:
1. In a large bowl, combine black beans, corn, red bell pepper, red onion, and cilantro.
2. In a small bowl, whisk together lime juice, olive oil, salt, and pepper.
3. Pour the dressing over the salad and toss to combine.
4. Garnish with avocado slices.
5. Serve chilled.

Nutritional Information (Per Serving):
- Calories: 380
- Protein: 14g
- Carbohydrates: 60g
- Fiber: 12g
- Sugars: 4g
- Fat: 10g
- Sodium: 480mg
- Potassium: 700mg

6.Vegetarian Lentil Soup
Prep Time:15minutes
Cooking Time:30minutes
Serving Size: 2
Ingredients:

- 1 cup dried green lentils, rinsed   1 onion, diced
- 2carrots, peeled and sliced
- 2 celery stalks, chopped
- 3 cloves garlic, minced
- 4 cups vegetable broth
- 1 can (14 oz) diced tomatoes
- 1 teaspoon cumin
- 1 teaspoon paprika
- 1/2 teaspoon turmeric
- Salt and pepper to taste
- Fresh parsley for garnish

Instructions:

1. In a large pot, sauté onion, carrots, celery, and garlic until softened.
2. Add dried lentils, vegetable broth, diced tomatoes, cumin, paprika, turmeric, salt, and pepper.
3. Bring to a boil, then reduce heat and simmer for 25-30 minutes.
4. Garnish with fresh parsley before serving.
5. Serve hot.

Nutritional Information (Per Serving):
- Calories: 350
- Protein: 18g
- Carbohydrates: 60g
- Fiber: 18g Sugars: 6g
- Fat: 5g
- Sodium: 900mg
- Potassium: 1200mg

7.Quinoa Salad with Chickpeas and Vegetables
Prep Time:15minutes
Cooking Time:20minutes
 Serving Size: 2
Ingredients:

- 1 cup quinoa, cooked
- 1 can (15 oz) chickpeas, drained and rinsed

- 1 cup cherry tomatoes, halved 1 cucumber, diced
- 1/2 red onion, finely chopped
- 1/4 cup feta cheese, crumbled
- 2 tablespoons olive oil
- 1 tablespoon balsamic vinegar
- Salt and pepper to taste
- Fresh herbs for garnish (optional)

Instructions:

1. In a large bowl, combine cooked quinoa, chickpeas, cherry tomatoes, cucumber, and red onion.

2. In a small bowl, whisk together olive oil, balsamic vinegar, salt, and pepper.

3. Pour the dressing over the quinoa mixture and toss to coat.

4. Sprinkle feta cheese on top.

5. Garnish with fresh herbs if desired.

6. Serve chilled.

Nutritional Information (Per Serving):

- Calories: 400
- Protein: 14g
- Carbohydrates: 55g
- Fiber: 10g
- Sugars: 6g
- Fat: 15g
- Sodium: 380mg
- Potassium: 650mg

Snacks

Choose a snack that combines protein and healthy fats. A handful of almonds with a piece of string cheese provides a satisfying and portable option to keep you satiated until your next meal.

1. Greek Yogurt and Berry Parfait

Prep Time: 10minutes
Cooking Time: 0minutes
Serving Size:
Ingredients:

- 1 cup Greek yogurt
- 1/2 cup mixed berries (strawberries, blueberries, raspberries)
- 1 tablespoon honey
- 1tablespoongranola

Instructions:

1. In a glass or bowl, layer Greek yogurt, mixed berries, and granola.
2. Drizzle honey over the top.
3. Repeat the layers if desired.
4. Serve chilled.

Nutritional Information (Per Serving):

- Calories: 250
- Protein: 15g
- Carbohydrates: 30g
- Fiber: 4g
- Sugars: 20g
- Fat: 8g
- Sodium: 80mg
- Potassium: 300mg

2.Whole Wheat Crackers with Hummus

Prep Time: 5minutes
Cooking Time: 0minutes
Serving Size: 10 crackers with 2 tablespoons hummus
Ingredients:

- whole wheat crackers
- 2 tablespoons hummus

Instructions:

1. Arrange whole wheat crackers on a plate.
2. Serve with hummus for dipping.
3. Enjoy!

Nutritional Information (Per Serving):

- Calories: 180
- Protein: 6g
- Carbohydrates: 25g

- Fiber: 4g
- Sugars: 1g
- Fat: 7g
- Sodium: 220mg
- Potassium: 150mg

3.Trail Mix
Prep Time: 5minutes
Cooking Time: 0minutes
Serving Size: 1/4 cup
Ingredients:
- 1/4 cup mixed nuts (almonds, walnuts, pistachios)
- 1 tablespoon dried cranberries
- 1 tablespoon dark chocolate chips

Instructions:
1. Combine mixed nuts, dried cranberries, and dark chocolate chips in a bowl.
2. Mix well and portion into 1/4 cup servings.
3. A perfect on-the-go snack.

Nutritional Information (Per Serving):
- Calories: 150
- Protein: 5g
- Carbohydrates: 10g
- Fiber: 2g
- Sugars: 5g
- Fat: 12g
- Sodium: 5mg
- Potassium: 150mg

4.Homemade Guacamole with Veggie Chips
Prep Time: 15minutes
Cooking Time: 10minutes
Serving Size: 1/2 cup guacamole with 1cup veggie chips
Ingredients:
- ripe avocados
- 1 tomato, diced
- 1/4 cup red onion, finely chopped
- 1/4 cup cilantro, chopped
- Juice of 1 lime
- Salt and pepper to taste
- 1 cup mixed veggie chips

Instructions:
1. In a bowl, mash avocados with a fork.
2. Add diced tomato, red onion, cilantro, lime juice, salt, and pepper. Mix well.
3. Serve with a side of mixed veggie chips.

Nutritional Information (Per Serving):

- Calories: 280
- Protein: 4g
- Carbohydrates: 20g
- Fiber: 8g
- Sugars: 3g
- Fat: 22g
- Sodium: 150mg
- Potassium: 600mg

5.Fruit Salad with Mint

Prep Time:15minutes

Cooking Time:0minutes

Serving Size: 1 cup

Ingredients:

. 1 cup mixed fruit (watermelon, pineapple, grapes, kiwi) Fresh mint leaves for garnish

Instructions:

1. Cut fruits into bite-sized pieces.
2. Combine in a bowl and garnish with fresh mint leaves.
3. A refreshing and healthy snack.

Nutritional Information (Per Serving):

- Calories: 80
- Protein: 1g
- Carbohydrates: 20g
- Fiber: 3g
- Sugars: 15g
- Fat: 0g
- Sodium: 0mg
- Potassium: 150mg

6.Cottage Cheese and Pineapple Bowl

Prep Time:10minutes

Cooking Time:0minutes

ServingSize:1cup

Ingredients:

. 1 cup low-fat cottage cheese
. 1 cup fresh pineapple chunks

Instructions:

1. Spoon cottage cheese into a bowl.

2. Top with fresh pineapple chunks.

3. An easy and protein-packed snack.

Nutritional Information (Per Serving):

- Calories: 220
- Protein: 26g
- Carbohydrates: 30g
- Fiber: 2g
- Sugars: 24g
- Fat: 2g
- Sodium: 460mg
- Potassium: 280mg

7. Roasted Chickpeas
Prep Time: 15minutes
Cooking Time: 25minutes
Serving Size: 1/2 cup
Ingredients:
- can (15 oz) chickpeas, drained and rinsed
- 1 tablespoon olive oil
- 1 teaspoon paprika
- 1/2 teaspoon cumin
- 1/2 teaspoon garlic powder
- Salt and pepper to taste

Instructions:
1. Preheat the oven to 400°F (200°C).
2. In a bowl, toss chickpeas with olive oil, paprika, cumin, garlic powder, salt, and pepper.
3. Spread chickpeas on a baking sheet.
4. Roast for 20-25 minutes, shaking the pan occasionally.
5. Allow to cool before serving.

Nutritional Information (Per Serving):
- Calories: 220
- Protein: 10g
- Carbohydrates: 30g
- Fiber: 7g
- Sugars: 5g
- Fat: 7g
- Sodium: 300mg
- Potassium: 280mg

Dinner

Keep dinner simple and flavorful with a stir-fry featuring tofu or lean protein, a variety of colorful vegetables, and a light soy-ginger sauce. Serve it over cauliflower rice for a lower-carb alternative.

1.Pasta Primavera with Grilled Chicken

Prep Time:15minutes
Cooking Time:20minutes
Serving Size: 1
Ingredients:

- oz whole wheat pasta
- 6 oz boneless, skinless chicken breast
- 1 cup mixed vegetables (zucchini, cherry tomatoes, bell peppers)
- 1 tablespoon olive oil
- 1/4 cup grated Parmesan cheese
- Fresh basil for garnish
- Salt and pepper to taste

Instructions:

1. Cook pasta according to package instructions.
2. Season chicken with salt and pepper and grill until cooked through.
3. In a skillet, sauté mixed vegetables with olive oil until tender.
4. Toss cooked pasta, grilled chicken, and sautéed vegetables together.
5. Garnish with grated Parmesan cheese and fresh basil.

Nutritional Information (Per Serving):

- Calories: 480
- Protein: 40g
- Carbohydrates: 40g
- Fiber: 8g
- Sugars: 4g
- Fat: 18g
- Sodium: 250mg
- Potassium: 750mg

2.Shrimp and Quinoa Bowl
Prep Time: 20minutes
Cooking Time: 15minutes
Serving Size: 1
Ingredients:

- 1/2 cup quinoa, cooked
- 8 oz shrimp, peeled and deveined
- 1 cup broccoli florets
- 1/2 cup cherry tomatoes, halved
- 1/4 cup feta cheese, crumbled
- 2 tablespoons olive oil
- Lemon wedges for serving
- Salt and pepper to taste

Instructions:

1. In a pan, heat olive oil over medium heat.
2. Add shrimp and cook until pink and opaque.
3. Steam broccoli until tender-crisp.
4. In a bowl, combine cooked quinoa, shrimp, steamed broccoli, cherry tomatoes, and feta cheese.
5. Drizzle with olive oil and season with salt and pepper.
6. Serve with lemon wedges.

Nutritional Information (Per Serving):

- Calories: 450
- Protein: 35g
- Carbohydrates: 35g
- Fiber: 5g
- Sugars: 3g
- Fat: 20g
- Sodium: 380mg
- Potassium: 620mg

3.Stuffed Bell Peppers with Turkey and Brown Rice
Prep Time:20minutes
Cooking Time:40minutes
ServingSize:2halves
Ingredients:

- 1/2 cup brown rice, cooked
- 1 lb ground turkey
- 4 bell peppers, halved and seeds removed
- 1 cup black beans, drained and rinsed
- 1 cup corn kernels
- 1 cup salsa
- 1 teaspoon cumin
- 1 teaspoon chili powder
- Salt and pepper to taste
- Shredded Monterey Jack cheese for topping

Instructions:

1. Preheat the oven to 375°F (190°C).
2. In a skillet, cook ground turkey until browned.
3. In a large bowl, mix cooked brown rice, browned turkey, black beans, corn, salsa, cumin, chili powder, salt, and pepper.
4. Stuff each bell pepper half with the turkey and rice mixture.
5. Top with shredded Monterey Jack cheese.
6. Bake for 30-40 minutes or until peppers are tender.

Nutritional Information (Per Serving):

- Calories: 430
- Protein: 30g
- Carbohydrates: 40g
- Fiber: 8g
- Sugars: 6g
- Fat: 18g
- Sodium: 520mg
- Potassium: 850mg

4.Chicken and Vegetable Stir-Fry with Brown Rice
Prep Time:15minutes
Cooking Time:20minutes
Serving Size:1
 Ingredients:

- 6 oz boneless, skinless chicken breast, thinly sliced
- 1 cup broccoli florets
- 1/2 cup snow peas
- 1 carrot, julienned
- 1/2 cup bell peppers, sliced
- 1 cup cooked brown rice
- 2 tablespoons low-sodium soy sauce
- 1 tablespoon sesame oil
- 1 tablespoon rice vinegar
- 1 teaspoon ginger, minced
- 1 clove garlic, minced
- Sesame seeds for garnish

Instructions:

1. In a wok or skillet, heat sesame oil over medium-high heat.
2. Add ginger and garlic, sauté for 1 minute.
3. Add chicken and stir-fry until cooked through.
4. Add broccoli, snow peas, carrot, and bell peppers. Stir-fry until vegetables are crisp-tender.
5. In a small bowl, mix soy sauce and rice vinegar. Pour over the stir-fry and toss to combine.
6. Serve over cooked brown rice and garnish with sesame seeds.

Nutritional Information (Per Serving):

- Calories: 420
- Protein: 35g
- Carbohydrates: 45g
- Fiber: 7g
- Sugars: 4g
- Fat: 15g
- Sodium: 600mg
- Potassium: 750mg

5.Vegetarian Lentil and Sweet Potato Curry
Prep Time:20minutes
Cooking Time:25minutes
Serving Size:1
Ingredients:

- . 1 cup lentils, cooked
- 1 sweet potato, diced
- 1 cup cauliflower florets
- 1 cup spinach leaves
- 1 can (14 oz) diced tomatoes
- 1 can (14 oz) coconut milk
- 1 onion, chopped
- 2 cloves garlic, minced
- 1 tablespoon curry powder
- 1 teaspoon turmeric
- Salt and pepper to taste
- Fresh cilantro for garnish

Instructions:

1. In a pot, sauté onion and garlic until softened.
2. Add diced sweet potato, cauliflower, lentils, diced tomatoes, coconut milk, curry powder, turmeric, salt, and pepper.
3. Simmer until sweet potatoes are tender.
4. Stir in spinach leaves and cook until wilted.
5. Garnish with fresh cilantro before serving.

Nutritional Information (Per Serving):

- Calories: 380
- Protein: 18g
- Carbohydrates: 55g
- Fiber: 15g
- Sugars: 8g
- Fat: 12g
- Sodium: 600mg
- Potassium: 1100mg

6.Mediterranean Quinoa Salad with Grilled Shrimp
PrepTime:15minutes
Cooking Time:15minutes
Serving Size: 1
Ingredients:

- 1/2 cup quinoa, cooked
- 8 oz shrimp, peeled and deveined
- 1 cup cherry tomatoes, halved
- 1/2 cucumber, diced

- 1/4 cup Kalamata olives, sliced
- 1/4 cup feta cheese, crumbled
- 2 tablespoons olive oil
- 1 tablespoon red wine vinegar
- Fresh oregano for garnish
- Salt and pepper to taste

Instructions:

1. Grill shrimp until pink and opaque.
2. In a bowl, combine cooked quinoa, grilled shrimp, cherry tomatoes, cucumber, Kalamata and olive and feta cheese
3. Drizzle with olive oil and red wine vinegar.
4. Toss to combine and garnish with fresh oregano.

Nutritional Information (Per Serving):

- Calories: 420
- Protein: 30g
- Carbohydrates: 40g
- Fiber: 7g
- Sugars: 4g
- Fat: 18g
- Sodium: 620mg
- Potassium: 650mg

7.Salmon and Asparagus Foil Packets

Prep Time:10minutes

Cooking Time:20minutes

Serving Size: 1

Ingredients:

- 6 oz salmon fillet
- 1 cup asparagus, trimmed
- 1 tablespoon olive oil
- 1 lemon, sliced
- Fresh dill for garnish
- Salt and pepper to taste

Instructions:

1. Preheat the oven to 400°F (200°C).
2. Place salmon fillet on a piece of foil.
3. Arrange asparagus around the salmon.
4. Drizzle with olive oil and season with salt and pepper.
5. Place lemon slices on top and fold the foil to create a packet.
6. Bake for 20 minutes or until salmon is cooked.
7. Garnish with fresh dill before serving.

Nutritional Information (Per Serving):

- Calories: 380
- Protein: 35g
- Carbohydrates: 10g
- Fiber: 4g
- Sugars: 2g
- Fat: 22g
- Sodium: 120mg
- Potassium: 900mg

CHAPTER 8: RECIPES FOR LOW CARB DAYS

Breakfast

Go for a protein-rich breakfast to kick off your low carb day. Consider a spinach and mushroom frittata with a side of avocado. This meal provides essential nutrients and healthy fats to fuel your morning.

1.Avocado and Egg Breakfast Bowl
Prep Time:5minutes
Cooking Time:5minutes
Serving Size: 1
Ingredients:

- 1 ripe avocado, halved and pitted

- 2 eggs

- Salt and pepper to taste

- Fresh herbs (optional)

Instructions:
1. Preheat the oven to 375°F (190°C).
2. Scoop out a small portion of the avocado flesh to create a well.
3. Crack an egg into each avocado half.
4. Season with salt and pepper.
5. Bake for 12-15 minutes or until the eggs are cooked to your liking.
6. Garnish with fresh herbs if desired.

Nutritional Information (Per Serving):
- Calories:32 0g
- Protein:5g
- Carbohydrate:8g
- Fiber: 7g
- Sugars: 1g
- Fat: 28g
- Sodium: 80mg
- Potassium: 700mg

2.Spinach and Feta Omelette
Prep Time: 10minutes
CookingTime:5minutes
ServingSize:1

Ingredients:

- eggs, beaten
- 1 cup fresh spinach, chopped
- 2 tablespoons feta cheese, crumbled
- Salt and pepper to taste
- 1 teaspoon olive oil

Instructions:

1. Heat olive oil in a non-stick skillet over medium heat.
2. Add chopped spinach and sauté until wilted.
3. Pour beaten eggs over the spinach.
4. Sprinkle feta cheese over the eggs.
5. Cook until the eggs are set, folding the omelette in half.
6. Season with salt and pepper.

Nutritional Information (Per Serving):

- Calories: 280
- Protein: 18g
- Carbohydrates: 3g
- Fiber: 1g
- Sugars: 1g
- Fat: 22g
- Sodium: 320mg
- Potassium: 450mg

3.Keto Chia Seed Pudding

Prep Time:5minutes (plus chilling time)

Cooking Time:0minutes

Serving Size: 1

Ingredients:

- tablespoons chia seeds
- 1/2 cup unsweetened almond milk
- 1/4teaspoon vanilla extract Stevia or erythritol to taste
- Fresh berries for topping

Instructions:

1. In a bowl, mix chia seeds, almond milk, vanilla extract, and sweetener.
2. Stir well and let it sit for at least 2 hours or overnight in the refrigerator.
3. Top with fresh berries before serving.

Nutritional Information (Per Serving):

- Calories: 180
- Protein: 5g
- Carbohydrates: 12g
- Fiber: 9g

- Sugars: 1g
- Fat: 13g
- Sodium: 80mg
- Potassium: 120mg

4.Low-Carb Egg Muffins

Prep Time:10minutes
Cooking Time:5minutes
Serving Size: 2 muffins
Ingredients:

- eggs
- 1/4 cup heavy cream
- 1/2 cup diced bell peppers
- 1/4 cup grated cheddar cheese
- Salt and pepper to taste

Instructions:

1. Preheat the oven to 350°F (175°C).
2. In a bowl, whisk together eggs and heavy cream.
3. Stir in diced bell peppers and grated cheddar cheese.
4. Season with salt and pepper.
5. Pour the mixture into greased muffin tins.
6. Bake for 20 minutes or until the eggs are set.

Nutritional Information (Per Serving):

- Calories: 280
- Protein: 14g
- Carbohydrates: 4g
- Fiber: 1g
- Sugars: 2g
- Fat: 22g
- Sodium: 260mg
- Potassium: 220mg

5.Almond Flour Pancakes

Prep Time:10minutes
Cooking Time:10minutes
Serving Size: 2 pancakes
Ingredients:

- 1 cup almond flour

- 2 eggs

- 1/4 cup unsweetened almond milk

- 1 tablespoon melted butter

- 1/2 teaspoon baking powder

- 1/2 teaspoon vanilla extract

- Pinch of salt

Instructions:

1. In a bowl, whisk together almond flour, eggs, almond milk, melted butter, baking powder, vanilla extract, and a pinch of salt.
2. Heat a griddle or skillet over medium heat.
3. Pour batter onto the griddle to form pancakes.
4. Cook until bubbles form on the surface, then flip and cook the other side.
5. Serve with sugar-free syrup if desired.

Nutritional Information (Per Serving):

- Calories: 320
- Protein: 12g
- Carbohydrates: 8g
- Fiber: 4g
- Sugars: 1g
- Fat: 28g
- Sodium: 320mg
- Potassium: 180mg

6.Cauliflower Hash Browns

Prep Time:15minutes

Cooking Time:15minutes

Serving Size: 3 hash browns

Ingredients:

- cups riced cauliflower
- 1 egg
- 1/4 cup almond flour
- 1/4 cup grated Parmesan cheese
- 1/2 teaspoon garlic powder
- Salt and pepper to taste

Instructions:

1. Preheat the oven to 400°F (200°C).
2. Mix riced cauliflower, egg, almond flour, grated Parmesan cheese, garlic powder, salt, and pepper in a bowl.
3. Form the mixture into small patties and place them on a baking sheet.
4. Bake for 15-20 minutes or until golden brown.

Nutritional Information (Per Serving):

- Calories: 180
- Protein: 10g
- Carbohydrates: 8g
- Fiber: 4g
- Sugars: 2g
- Fat: 12g
- Sodium: 320mg
- Potassium: 450mg

7.Smoked Salmon and Cream Cheese Roll-Ups

Prep Time:10minutes

Cooking Time:0minutes

Serving Size: 2 roll-ups

Ingredients:

- oz smoked salmon
- 2 tablespoons cream cheese
- 1 tablespoon capers
- Fresh dill for garnish

Instructions:

1. Lay out the smoked salmon slices.
2. Spread cream cheese on each slice.
3. Sprinkle capers over the cream cheese.
4. Roll up the smoked salmon slices.
5. Garnish with fresh dill.

Nutritional Information (Per Serving):

- Calories: 220
- Protein: 18g
- Carbohydrates: 2g
- Fiber: 0g
- Sugars: 1g
- Fat: 16g
- Sodium: 820mg
- Potassium: 350mg

Lunch

Keep lunch light but satisfying with a grilled chicken or shrimp Caesar salad. Load up on leafy greens, lean protein, and a moderate amount of Caesar dressing for flavor.

1.Eggplant Lasagna Roll-Ups
Prep Time:20minutes
Cooking Time:30minutes
Serving Size: 2 roll-ups
Ingredients:

- 1 medium eggplant, thinly sliced lengthwise

- 1 cup ricotta cheese

- 1/2 cup marinara sauce (sugar-free)

- 1 cup shredded mozzarella cheese

- 1 tablespoon olive oil

- Fresh basil for garnish

- Salt and pepper to taste

Instructions:
1. Preheat the oven to 375°F (190°C).
2. Grill the eggplant slices until tender.
3. In a bowl, mix ricotta cheese, salt, and pepper.
4. Spread a thin layer of marinara sauce on each eggplant slice.
5. Spoon the ricotta mixture onto each slice and roll them up.
6. Place the roll-ups in a baking dish, top with mozzarella, and bake until cheese is melted and bubbly.
7. Garnish with fresh basil before serving.

Nutritional Information (Per Serving):
- Calories: 280
- Protein: 16g
- Carbohydrates: 8g
- Fiber: 4g
- Sugars: 3g
- Fat: 18g
- Sodium: 420mg
- Potassium: 550mg

2.Zucchini Noodles with Pesto and Cherry Tomatoes

Prep Time:15minutes

CookingTime:5minute

Serving Size: 1

Ingredient

- medium zucchinis, spiralized
- 1/4 cup pesto sauce
- 1/2 cup cherry tomatoes, halved
- 1 tablespoon pine nuts 1tablespoon olive oil
- Fresh basil for garnish
- Salt and pepper to taste

Instructions:

1. Spiralize the zucchinis to form noodles.
2. In a pan, heat olive oil and sauté zucchini noodles until tender.
3. Add pesto sauce and cherry tomatoes, toss until combined.
4. Toast pine nuts in a dry pan until golden.
5. Garnish the noodles with toasted pine nuts and fresh basil.
6. Season with salt and pepper.

Nutritional Information (Per Serving):

- Calories: 250
- Protein: 6g
- Carbohydrates: 10g
- Fiber: 3g
- Sugars: 4g
- Fat: 20g
- Sodium: 320mg
- Potassium: 780mg

3.Turkey and Avocado Lettuce Wraps

Prep Time:10minutes

Cooking Time:0minutes

ServingSize:2wraps

Ingredients:

- 8 large lettuce leaves (butter or iceberg)
- 8 oz ground turkey, cooked
- 1 avocado, sliced
- 1/2 cup cherry tomatoes, halved
- 1/4 cup red onion, finely chopped
- Greek yogurt (optional)
- Cilantro for garnish
- Salt and pepper to taste

Instructions:

1. Lay out lettuce leaves.
2. Fill each leaf with cooked ground turkey.
3. Top with avocado slices, cherry tomatoes, and red onion.

4. Drizzle with Greek yogurt if desired.
5. Garnish with fresh cilantro.
6. Season with salt and pepper.

Nutritional Information (Per Serving):

- Calories: 280
- Protein: 20g
- Carbohydrates: 8g
- Fiber: 4g
- Sugars: 2g
- Fat: 18g
- Sodium: 320mg
- Potassium: 650mg

4.Spinach and Feta Stuffed Chicken Breast

Prep Time:20minutes
CookingTime:25minutes
Serving Size: 1
Ingredients:

- 6 oz chicken breast
- 1 cup fresh spinach, chopped
- 2 tablespoons feta cheese, crumbled
- 1 clove garlic, minced
- 1 teaspoon olive oil
- Lemon juice for drizzling
- Salt and pepper to taste

Instructions:

1. Preheat the oven to 375°F (190°C).
2. In a pan, sauté chopped spinach and minced garlic in olive oil until wilted.
3. Make a pocket in the chicken breast and stuff with sautéed spinach and feta.
4. Season the chicken with salt and pepper.
5. Bake until the chicken is cooked through.
6. Drizzle with fresh lemon juice before serving.

Nutritional Information (Per Serving):

- Calories: 290
- Protein: 30g
- Carbohydrates: 2g
- Fiber: 1g
- Sugars: 0g
- Fat: 18g
- Sodium: 380mg
- Potassium: 500mg

5.Cauliflower and Broccoli Gratin

Prep Time:20minutes

Cooking Time:30minutes

ServingSize:1

Ingredients:

- Cup cauliflower
- 1 cup broccoli florets
- 1/2cupcheddar cheese, shredded
- 1/4 cup heavy cream
- 1 tablespoon butter
- 1clove garlic, minced
- Salt and pepper taste
- Fresh parsley for garnish

Instructions:

1. Preheat the oven to 375°F (190°C).
2. Steam cauliflower and broccoli until tender.
3. In a saucepan, melt butter and sauté minced garlic until fragrant.
4. Stir in heavy cream and shredded cheddar cheese until smooth.
5. Place steamed cauliflower and broccoli in a baking dish.
6. Pour the cheese sauce over the vegetables.
7. Bake until the top is golden and bubbly.
8. Garnish with fresh parsley.

Nutritional Information (Per Serving):

- Calories: 290
- Protein: 12g
- Carbohydrates: 8g
- Fiber: 3g
- Sugars: 3g
- Fat: 22g
- Sodium: 320mg
- Potassium: 680mg

6.Salmon and Asparagus Foil Packets

Prep Time:15minutes

Cooking Time:20minutes
Serving Size: 1
Ingredients:

- 6 oz salmon fillet
- 1 cup asparagus, trimmed
- 1 tablespoon olive oil
- 1 tablespoon lemon juice
- 1 teaspoon Dijon mustard
- Fresh dill for garnish
- Salt and pepper to taste

Instructions:

1. Preheat the oven to 400°F (200°C).
2. In a bowl, whisk together olive oil, lemon juice, and Dijon mustard.
3. Place salmon and asparagus on a large piece of foil.
4. Drizzle the olive oil mixture over the salmon and asparagus.
5. Seal the foil packet and bake until salmon is cooked.
6. Garnish with fresh dill.
7. Season with salt and pepper.

Nutritional Information (Per Serving):

- Calories: 320g
- Protein: 25g
- Carbohydrates: 6g
- Fiber: 3g
- Sugars: 2g
- Fat: 22g
- Sodium: 380mg
- Potassium: 750mg

7.Shrimp Stir-Fry with Vegetables
Prep Time:20minutes
Cooking Time:15minutes
Serving Size: 1
Ingredients:

- 6 oz shrimp, peeled and deveined
- 1 cup broccoli florets
- 1/2 bell pepper, sliced
- 1/2 cup snow peas
- 1 tablespoon soy sauce (low-sodium)
- 1 tablespoon sesame oil
- 1 teaspoon ginger, minced
- 2 cloves garlic, minced
- Green onions for garnish

Instructions:

1. In a wok or pan, heat sesame oil and sauté ginger and garlic until fragrant.

2. Add shrimp and cook until they turn pink.
3. Stir in broccoli, bell pepper, and snow peas.
4. Pour in soy sauce and toss until vegetables are tender.
5. Garnish with chopped green onions.

Nutritional Information (Per Serving):

- Calories: 280
- Protein: 24g
- Carbohydrates: 10g
- Fiber: 4g
- Sugars: 4g
- Fat: 16g
- Sodium: 780mg
- Potassium: 550mg

Snacks

Choose a snack that aligns with your low carb goals. A serving of sliced cucumber with hummus offers a crunchy and flavorful option that keeps carb intake in check.

1.Cucumber and Cream Cheese Roll-Ups
Prep Time:10minutes
Cooking Time:0minutes
Serving Size: 4 roll-ups
Ingredients:

- 1large cucumber

- 4 oz cream cheese

- Smoked almon (optional)

- Fresh dill for garnish

- salt and pepper to taste

Instructions:
1. Slice the cucumber into thin strips using a peeler.
2. Spread a thin layer of cream cheese on each cucumber strip.
3. Optionally, add a strip of smoked salmon on top.
4. Roll up the cucumber strips and secure with toothpicks.
5. Garnish with fresh dill and season with salt and pepper.

Nutritional Information (Per Serving):
- Calories: 90
- Protein: 3g
- Fiber: 1g
- Sugars: 2g
- Fat: 7g
- Sodium: 120mg
- Potassium: 240mg

2.Avocado and Bacon Deviled Eggs
Prep Time:15minutes
Cooking Time:10minutes
ServingSize:2halves
Ingredients:
- 4 hard-boiled eggs, halved
- 1 ripe avocado

- 2 slices cooked bacon, crumbled
- Chives for garnish
- Salt and pepper to taste

Instructions:

1. Scoop out the yolks from the halved eggs.
2. Mash the yolks with ripe avocado until smooth.
3. Stir in crumbled bacon and season with salt and pepper.
4. Spoon the mixture back into the egg whites.
5. Garnish with chopped chives.

Nutritional Information (Per Serving):

- Calories: 150
- Protein: 7g
- Carbohydrates: 5g
- Fiber: 3g
- Sugars: 0g
- Fat: 11g
- Sodium: 160mg
- Potassium: 380mg

3.Eggplant Pizza Bites
Prep Time:20minutes
Cooking Time:15minutes
Serving Size: 4 pieces
Ingredients:

- 1 large eggplant, sliced into rounds
- 1/2 cup sugar-free marinara sauce
- 1 cup shredded mozzarella cheese
- Cherry tomatoes, sliced olives, and basil for topping
- Olive oil for drizzling
- Italian seasoning

Instructions:

1. Preheat the oven to 375°F (190°C).
2. Place eggplant rounds on a baking sheet.
3. Spread marinara sauce on each round.
4. Sprinkle shredded mozzarella and add desired toppings.

5. Drizzle with olive oil and sprinkle with Italian seasoning.

6. Bake until the cheese is melted and bubbly.

Nutritional Information (Per Serving):

- Calories: 120
- Protein: 5g
- Carbohydrates: 10g
- Fiber: 5g
- Sugars: 4g
- Fat: 7g
- Sodium: 160mg
- Potassium: 480mg

4.Cheese and Olive Skewers

Prep Time:10minutes

Cooking Time:0minutes

Serving Size: 4 skewers

Ingredients:

- 1 cup mozzarella balls

- Cherry tomatoes

- Green olives

- Basil leaves

- Balsamic glaze for drizzling

Instructions:

1. Thread mozzarella balls, cherry tomatoes, green olives, and basil onto skewers.

2. Arrange on a serving platter.

3. Drizzle with balsamic glaze before serving.

Nutritional Information (Per Serving):

- Calories: 120
- Protein: 6g
- Carbohydrates: 3g
- Fiber: 1g
- Sugars: 1g
- Fat: 9g
- Sodium: 180mg
- Potassium: 240mg

5.Greek Cucumber Cups

Prep Time:15minutes
Cooking Time:0minutes
Serving Size: 4 cups
Ingredients:
- large cucumbers
- 1 cup cherry tomatoes, diced
- 1/2 cup feta cheese, crumbled
- Kalamata olives, sliced
- Red onion, finely chopped
- Tzatziki sauce for topping

Instructions:
1. Peel strips from cucumbers to create a striped pattern.
2. Slice cucumbers into thick rounds.
3. Hollow out the center of each cucumber round.
4. Fill cucumber cups with diced tomatoes, feta, olives, and red onion.
5. Top with a dollop of tzatziki sauce.

Nutritional Information (Per Serving):
- Calories: 90
- Protein: 5g
- Carbohydrates: 8g
- Fiber: 2g
- Sugars: 4g
- Fat: 5g
- Sodium: 240mg
- Potassium: 380mg

6.Spinach and Artichoke Dip
Prep Time:20minutes
Cooking Time:20minutes
Serving Size: 1/4 cup dip with veggie sticks
Ingredients:
- 1 cup frozen chopped spinach, thawed and drained
- 1 cup artichoke hearts, chopped
- 1/2 cup mayonnaise
- 1/2 cup sour cream
- 1 cup shredded Parmesan cheese
- 1 clove garlic, minced
- Assorted vegetable sticks for dipping

Instructions:
1. Preheat the oven to 375°F (190°C).
   In a bowl, mix together spinach, artichoke hearts, mayonnaise, sour cream, Parmesan cheese,

and   minced garlic.

2. Transfer the mixture to a baking dish.

3. Bake until hot and bubbly.

4. Serve with assorted vegetable sticks.

Nutritional Information (Per Serving):

- · Calories: 140
- · Protein: 5g
- · Carbohydrates: 4g
- · Fiber: 2g
- · Sugars: 1g
- · Fat: 12g
- · Sodium: 280mg
- · Potassium: 300mg

7.Broccoli and Cheddar Bites
Prep Time:15minutes
Cooking
Time:15minutes
ServingSize:4bites
Ingredients:

- • 1 cup steamed broccoli, finely chopped

- • 1 cup sharp cheddar cheese, shredded

- • 1/2 cup almond flour

- • 2 eggs

- • 1 teaspoon garlic powder

- • Salt and pepper to taste

- • Greek yogurt for dipping

Instructions:

1. Preheat the oven to 400°F (200°C).
2. In a bowl, combine chopped broccoli, cheddar cheese, almond flour, eggs, garlic powder, salt, and pepper.
3. Form the mixture into bite-sized balls and place on a baking sheet.
4. Bake until golden brown and cooked through.
5. Serve with a side of Greek yogurt for dipping.

Nutritional Information (Per Serving):

- · Calories: 140

- Protein: 8g
- Carbohydrates: 4g
- Fiber: 2g
- Sugars: 1g
- Fat: 10g
- Sodium: 180mg
- Potassium: 250mg

Dinner

Wrap up your low carb day with a grilled steak or vegetable stir-fry featuring non-starchy veggies like bell peppers, broccoli, and asparagus. Pair it with a side of sautéed spinach for added nutrients.

Designing daily meal plans for different carb cycling phases is about variety, balance, and enjoyment. Experiment with ingredients and flavors to find combinations that suit your taste preferences while aligning with your carb cycling goals.

1.Grilled Lemon Herb Chicken
PrepTime:15minutes
CookingTime:20minutes
Serving Size:1 chicken
breast **Ingredients:**
- boneless, skinless chicken breasts
- 2 tablespoons olive oil
- 1 lemon (juiced)
- 2 cloves garlic (minced)
- 1 teaspoon dried oregano
- 1 teaspoon dried thyme
- Salt and pepper to taste

Instructions:
1. Preheat the grill to medium-high heat.
2. In a bowl, mix olive oil, lemon juice, minced garlic, oregano, thyme, salt, and pepper.
3. Marinate chicken breasts in the mixture for at least 10 minutes.
4. Grill chicken for 10-12 minutes per side or until fully cooked.
5. Let it rest for a few minutes before serving.

Nutritional Information (Per Serving):
- Calories: 300
- Protein: 30g
- Carbohydrates: 2g
- Fiber: 1g
- Sugars: 0g
- Fat: 18g
- Sodium: 120mg
- Potassium: 400mg

2.Eggplant Lasagna
Prep Time:30minutes
Cooking Time:40minutes
Serving Size: 1 slice
Ingredients:

- 1 large eggplant, sliced

- 1 lb ground beef or turkey

- 1 cup ricotta cheese

- 1 cup mozzarella cheese, shredded

- 1 cup marinara sauce

- 2 tablespoons olive oil

- 1 teaspoon dried basil

- Salt and pepper to taste

Instructions:
1. Preheat the oven to 375°F (190°C).
2. Grill or bake eggplant slices until tender.
3. In a skillet, brown ground meat in olive oil.
4. In a baking dish, layer eggplant, meat, ricotta, mozzarella, marinara, and basil.
5. Repeat layers and bake for 25-30 minutes.

Nutritional Information (Per Serving):
- Calories: 320
- Protein: 20g
- Carbohydrates: 12g
- Fiber: 5g
- Sugars: 6g
- Fat: 22g
- Sodium: 300mg
- Potassium: 700mg

3.Shrimp and Avocado Salad
Prep Time:15minutes
Cooking Time:5minutes

Serving Size: 1 salad

Ingredients:

- lb shrimp, peeled and deveined
- 2 avocados, sliced
- 1 cup cherry tomatoes, halved
- 1 cucumber, sliced
- 1/4 cup feta cheese, crumbled
- 2 tablespoons olive oil
- 1 tablespoon balsamic vinegar
- Salt and pepper to taste

Instructions:

1. Season shrimp with salt and pepper.
2. In a skillet, sauté shrimp in olive oil until cooked.
3. In a bowl, combine shrimp, avocados, cherry tomatoes, cucumber, and feta.
4. Drizzle with balsamic vinegar.

Nutritional Information (Per Serving):

- Calories: 350
- Protein: 25g
- Carbohydrates: 15g
- Fiber: 8g
- Sugars: 4g
- Fat: 24g
- Sodium: 400mg
- Potassium: 800mg

4.Zoodle Alfredo with Chicken
Prep Time:20minutes
Cooking
Time:15minutes
ServingSize:1cup
Ingredients:

- zucchinis, spiralized into noodles
- 1 lb chicken breast, sliced
- 1 cup broccoli florets

- 1cup Alfredo sauce (made with cream, Parmesan, and butter)
- 1tablespoons olive oil
- cloves garlic (minced)
- Salt and pepper to taste

Instructions:

1. In a pan, sauté sliced chicken in olive oil until cooked.
2. Add minced garlic and broccoli, cook until tender.
3. Add zucchini noodles and Alfredo sauce, toss until heated.
4. Season with salt and pepper.

Nutritional Information (Per Serving):

- Calories: 400
- Protein: 30g
- Carbohydrates: 10g
- Fiber: 3g
- Sugars: 2g
- Fat: 28g
- Sodium: 300mg
- Potassium: 700mg

5.Cabbage and Ground Beef Stir-Fry
Prep Time:15minutes
Cooking Time:20minutes
Serving Size: 1 cup
Ingredients:

- 1 lb ground beef

- 1 small cabbage, shredded

- 1 bell pepper, sliced

- 1 onion, sliced

- 2 tablespoons soy sauce

- 1 tablespoon sesame oil

- 1 teaspoon ginger (minced)

- 2 cloves garlic (minced)

- Salt and pepper to taste

Instructions:

1. In a wok or skillet, brown ground beef.
2. Add minced ginger and garlic, stir until fragrant.
3. Add shredded cabbage, bell pepper, and onion. Cook until vegetables are tender.
4. Stir in soy sauce and sesame oil. Season with salt and pepper.

Nutritional Information (Per Serving):
- Calories: 320
- Protein: 25g
- Carbohydrates: 10g
- Fiber: 4g
- Sugars: 6g
- Fat: 20g
- Sodium: 600mg
- Potassium: 700mg

6.Turkey and Vegetable Skewers
Prep Time:15minutes
Cooking Time:15minutes
Serving Size: 2 skewers
Ingredients:

- lb turkey breast, cut into chunks
- Bell peppers, cherry tomatoes, and red onions (for skewers)
- 2 tablespoons olive oil
- 1 teaspoon paprika
- 1/2 teaspoon cumin
- Salt and pepper to taste

Instructions:
1. Preheat the grill to medium-high heat.
2. Thread turkey and vegetables onto skewers.
3. In a bowl, mix olive oil, paprika, cumin, salt, and pepper.
4. Brush the skewers with the mixture and grill for 10-15 minutes.

Nutritional Information (Per Serving):
- Calories: 280
- Protein: 30g
- Carbohydrates: 8g
- Fiber: 3g
- Sugars: 4g
- Fat: 14g
- Sodium: 300mg

- Potassium: 600mg

7.Turkey and Zucchini Skillet
Prep Time:15minutes
Cooking Time:20minutes
Serving Size: 1 cup
Ingredients:

- 1 lb ground turkey
- 2 zucchinis, diced
- 1 bell pepper, diced
- 1 cup cherry tomatoes, halved
- 2 tablespoons olive oil
- 2 cloves garlic (minced)
- 1 teaspoon Italian seasoning
- Salt and pepper to taste

Instructions:

1. In a skillet, brown ground turkey in olive oil.
2. Add minced garlic, diced zucchini, bell pepper, and cherry tomatoes.
3. Cook until vegetables are tender.
4. Season with Italian seasoning, salt, and pepper.

Nutritional Information (Per Serving):

- Calories: 250
- Protein: 25g
- Carbohydrates: 8g
- Fiber: 2g
- Sugars: 4g
- Fat: 15g
- Sodium: 80mg
- Potassium: 600mg

CHAPTER 9: MAXIMIZING WORKOUTS WITH CARB CYCLING

Pre- and Post-Workout Nutrition Strategies

Maximizing your workouts through strategic pre- and post-workout nutrition is a cornerstone of effective carb cycling. These strategies not only optimize your energy levels but also support recovery, ensuring that your body is primed for peak performance during exercise.

Pre-Workout Nutrition:

Fueling your body before a workout is akin to filling up your car's gas tank before a long journey – it ensures a smooth and efficient ride. For high and moderate carb days:

Timing is Key: Consume a balanced meal containing a mix of carbohydrates, protein, and a small amount of healthy fats about 2-3 hours before your workout. This allows your body to digest and utilize the nutrients for sustained energy.

Carb Emphasis: Prioritize complex carbohydrates such as whole grains, sweet potatoes, or fruits. These provide a gradual release of glucose, sustaining your energy levels throughout the workout. Combine them with a lean protein source for muscle support.

Hydration Matters: Don't forget the importance of hydration. Pre-workout hydration sets the stage for optimal performance. Aim to drink water consistently throughout the day and consider sipping on water infused with electrolytes for added hydration support.

For low carb days:

Moderate Protein Intake: Focus on a protein-rich pre-workout snack or meal. Include sources like lean chicken, eggs, or Greek yogurt. While carbs are limited, a moderate protein intake helps support muscle function during exercise.

Include Healthy Fats: Incorporate healthy fats, such as avocados or nuts, for sustained energy. While the emphasis is on protein and healthy fats, a small amount of low-glycemic carbs can be included for those who find it beneficial.

Post-Workout Nutrition:

After a workout, your body craves replenishment and recovery. Tailoring your post-workout nutrition to the carb cycling phase ensures you optimize these crucial aspects:

Carb and Protein Combo: Consume a combination of carbohydrates and protein within the first hour post-exercise. This replenishes glycogen stores and provides amino acids for muscle repair. Opt for a banana with a protein shake, whole grain toast with peanut butter, or Greek yogurt with berries. **Adjusting Carb Intake:** On high carb days, you can afford a more substantial carb intake postworkout to fully replenish glycogen stores. On moderate carb days, maintain a balanced ratio of carbs to protein, and on low carb days, focus more on protein with a smaller amount of carbs.

Hydrate: Rehydrate with water or a sports drink containing electrolytes. Sweating during exercise leads to fluid loss, and replenishing electrolytes aids in optimal recovery.

Strategic pre- and post-workout nutrition sets the stage for improved performance, faster recovery, and better overall fitness results. Adapting these strategies to different carb cycling phases ensures that your body receives the specific nutrients it needs at the right time.

Adapting Carb Cycling to Fitness Goals

Carb cycling is a versatile tool that can be adapted to various fitness goals, whether you aim to lose weight, build muscle, enhance athletic performance, or achieve overall wellness. Tailoring your carb cycling approach to your specific objectives ensures that your nutritional plan aligns with your fitness journey.

Weight Loss:

Caloric Deficit: For weight loss goals, creating a caloric deficit is fundamental. On low and moderate carb days, focus on lean protein, healthy fats, and a variety of non-starchy vegetables. These nutrient dense options help control calorie intake while providing essential vitamins and minerals.

Strategic Carb Timing: Emphasize carb intake around workouts to support energy levels. High carb days can be strategically placed on more active days, ensuring that your body has the fuel it needs during intense exercise.

Mindful Eating: Incorporate mindful eating practices to prevent overconsumption. Pay attention to hunger and fullness cues, and savor each meal. This mindful approach fosters a healthy relationship with food and supports weight loss efforts.

Muscle Building:

Protein Prioritization: Protein is paramount for muscle building. Ensure an adequate protein intake on all carb cycling days, with a slight emphasis on high-quality protein sources on low and moderate carb days. This supports muscle repair and growth.

Strategic Carb Loading: Schedule high carb days on intense training days, especially those focused on resistance training. The increased carbohydrate intake provides the energy necessary for challenging workouts and aids in muscle glycogen replenishment.

Nutrient Timing: Pay attention to nutrient timing, especially around workouts. Consume a balanced meal with a mix of protein and carbs before exercising to provide the necessary fuel. Post-workout, prioritize a combination of protein and carbs to support recovery.

Athletic Performance:

Carb Loading for Endurance: Athletes engaging in endurance activities benefit from carb loading on specific days. This involves consuming a higher percentage of carbohydrates in the days leading up to a competition or intense training session. This maximizes glycogen stores for prolonged energy. **Periodization:** Implement carb cycling in a periodized manner, aligning high carb days with more demanding training phases. Adjust carb intake based on the intensity and duration of your athletic pursuits, ensuring that your body has the fuel required for peak performance.

Hydration and Electrolytes: Prioritize hydration, especially for endurance athletes. Alongside carb cycling, maintain optimal fluid balance and consider incorporating electrolyte-rich foods or beverages to prevent dehydration during prolonged exercise.

Overall Wellness:

Balanced Nutrition: Regardless of specific fitness goals, prioritize balanced nutrition. Ensure a variety of fruits, vegetables, lean proteins, and healthy fats in your diet. This provides a broad spectrum of nutrients essential for overall health and well-being.

Flexibility and Sustainability: Approach carb cycling with flexibility and sustainability in mind. It's essential that your nutritional plan is adaptable to different phases of life, allowing you to maintain a healthy lifestyle without feeling overly restricted.

Regular Assessments: Regularly assess your progress and adjust your carb cycling approach as needed. Listen to your body, monitor energy levels, and make modifications based on how your fitness goals evolve over time.

Adapting carb cycling to your fitness goals requires a thoughtful and personalized approach. Whether your focus is weight loss, muscle building, athletic performance, or overall wellness, tailoring your nutritional plan ensures that carb cycling becomes a valuable ally on your fitness journey.

Enhancing Energy Levels for Exercise

Sustained energy levels are crucial for maximizing the effectiveness of your workouts. Whether you're engaging in high intensity training or endurance activities, optimizing energy levels through carb cycling can significantly impact your performance and overall exercise experience.

Strategic Carb Timing:

Pre-Workout Carb Intake: On high carb days, strategically time your carbohydrate intake to align with your workout. Consuming complex carbohydrates 1-2 hours before exercise ensures that your body has a readily available source of energy. This is particularly beneficial for high-intensity and prolonged workouts.

Targeted Carb Intake: For specific workouts or training phases, consider implementing targeted carb intake. This involves consuming a moderate amount of carbs around your workout to provide an energy boost without affecting overall carb cycling goals. This approach can enhance performance without disrupting your carb cycling routine.

Metabolic Flexibility:

Training Your Body: Carb cycling enhances metabolic flexibility, allowing your body to efficiently switch between using carbohydrates and fats for fuel. This flexibility is valuable for endurance athletes and those engaged in activities that demand varied energy sources.

Adaptation to Low Carb Days: Embrace the adaptation process on low carb days. Initially, your body may take time to adjust to lower carbohydrate intake. However, over time, it becomes more adept at utilizing stored fat for energy, leading to improved endurance and sustained energy levels during workouts.

Hydration and Electrolytes:

Water Intake: Proper hydration is fundamental for maintaining energy levels. Dehydration can lead to fatigue and decreased exercise performance. Aim to drink water consistently throughout the day, adjusting your intake based on activity level and climate.

Electrolyte Balance: Especially during intense or prolonged exercise, maintaining electrolyte balance is crucial. Incorporate electrolyte-rich foods or beverages, such as sports drinks or coconut water, to prevent imbalances that can contribute to fatigue and cramping.

Individualized Approach

Listen to Your Body: Pay attention to how your body responds to different carb cycling phases. If you find that your energy levels are consistently low during workouts, consider adjusting the timing and composition of your meals to better suit your needs.

Experimentation: Carb cycling is not a one-size-fits-all approach. It may require some experimentation to find the right balance for your body. Be open to making adjustments based on your energy levels, workout intensity, and overall well-being.

Enhancing energy levels for exercise through carb cycling involves a thoughtful and individualized approach. By strategically timing carb intake, promoting metabolic flexibility, and prioritizing hydration, you can optimize your body's performance and make the most of each workout, contributing to your overall fitness success.

CHAPTER10: OVERCOMING CHALLENGES AND COMMON MISTAKE

Addressing Potential Side Effects

Embarking on a carb cycling journey can be transformative, but like any dietary adjustment, it may come with potential side effects. Understanding and addressing these side effects is crucial to ensure a positive and sustainable experience.

Low Energy Levels:

Cause: Low energy levels often arise during the adjustment phase as the body transitions to using stored fat for energy. Additionally, inadequate calorie intake, especially on low carb days, can contribute to fatigue.

Solution: Gradually introduce carb cycling to allow the body to adapt. Ensure that you're meeting overall calorie needs, especially on high activity days. Consider adjusting the timing and distribution of macronutrients to better align with your energy demands.

Digestive Issues:

Cause: Changes in dietary fiber intake, particularly an abrupt increase in fiber-rich foods, can lead to digestive issues such as bloating or constipation.

Solution: Increase fiber gradually to allow the digestive system to adapt. Hydrate well to support proper digestion. Include a variety of fiber sources, such as fruits, vegetables, and whole grains, for a well-rounded approach.

Mood Swings:

Cause: Carb cycling can influence serotonin levels, impacting mood. Additionally, drastic fluctuations in blood sugar levels may contribute to mood swings.

Solution: Prioritize complex carbohydrates to provide a steady release of glucose. Include foods rich in serotonin precursors, such as turkey, nuts, and seeds. Ensure consistent meal timing to prevent extreme blood sugar fluctuations.

Sleep Disturbances:

Cause: Changes in dietary patterns, especially in carb intake close to bedtime, may affect sleep. Disruptions in blood sugar levels can impact sleep quality.

Solution: Limit high carb intake close to bedtime and opt for a balanced evening meal. Incorporate sleep-promoting foods like nuts, seeds, and dairy. Establish a consistent sleep routine to enhance overall sleep quality.

Cravings

Cause: Restricting certain foods on low carb days may trigger cravings, especially for high-carb or sugary items.

Solution: Allow for flexibility in your diet to accommodate occasional cravings. Choose nutrient-dense alternatives for satisfying sweet cravings, such as fruits or dark chocolate in moderation.

Understanding and addressing potential side effects is a crucial aspect of a successful carb cycling journey. By being mindful of your body's responses and making adjustments as needed, you can navigate these challenges effectively and ensure a positive experience.

Troubleshooting Plateaus

Experiencing plateaus during a carb cycling journey is not uncommon. Plateaus can be frustrating, but they are also opportunities for assessment and refinement. Here's how to troubleshoot plateaus and keep your progress on track:

Reassess Your Caloric Intake:

Issue: Plateaus can occur if your body has adapted to a consistent caloric intake. Over time, metabolic adjustments may lead to a plateau in weight loss or muscle gain.

Solution: Reassess your caloric needs. If you've been in a caloric deficit for an extended period, consider a brief maintenance or surplus phase before returning to a deficit. This can help reset your metabolism.

Evaluate Macronutrient Ratios:
Issue: Sticking to the same macronutrient ratios for an extended period may contribute to plateaus. Your body might adapt to the consistent intake, affecting progress.

Solution: Experiment with adjusting macronutrient ratios. For example, slightly increase or decrease your carbohydrate intake on different days. This variation can stimulate changes in energy expenditure and metabolism.

Review Workout Intensity:

Issue: Your body adapts to exercise routines over time, potentially leading to a plateau in performance and results.

Solution: Introduce variety into your workouts. Increase intensity, incorporate new exercises, or modify your training split. Periodically challenge your body to prevent adaptation and enhance overall fitness.

Consider Stress Levels:
Issue: Elevated stress levels can hinder progress by affecting hormones associated with metabolism and

recovery.

Solution: Prioritize stress management techniques such as meditation, yoga, or deep breathing exercises.

Ensure sufficient rest and recovery to support your body's adaptation to training.

Monitor Sleep Quality:

Issue: Inadequate or poor-quality sleep can impact metabolism, recovery, and overall well-being, contributing to plateaus.

Solution: Establish a consistent sleep routine and prioritize sufficient sleep. Create a conducive sleep environment, limit screen time before bed, and address any factors affecting sleep quality.

Stay Hydrated:

Issue: Dehydration can impact physical performance and energy levels, potentially leading to plateaus.

Solution: Ensure adequate hydration throughout the day. Consider factors such as climate, activity level, and individual hydration needs. Proper hydration supports overall health and can positively influence performance.

Track Non-Scale Victories:

Issue: Overemphasis on the scale can be demotivating, especially during plateaus.

Solution: Track non-scale victories such as changes in body composition, improvements in strength or endurance, and enhanced energy levels. Celebrate these achievements as indicators of overall progress. Plateaus are a natural part of any fitness journey. By adopting a proactive and strategic approach, you can navigate plateaus successfully and continue making progress toward your goals.

Staying Consistent with Carb Cycling

Consistency is key in any dietary approach, and carb cycling is no exception. Maintaining a consistent and sustainable carb cycling practice ensures long-term success. Here's how to stay committed to your carb cycling journey:

Plan and Prep Meals:

Establish a Routine: Plan your meals in advance and establish a routine that aligns with your carb cycling phases. Knowing what you'll eat and when helps create a sense of structure.

Meal Prep: Prepare meals in batches, especially for days when time may be limited. Having prepped meals reduces the likelihood of reaching for less healthy options due to convenience.

Set Realistic Goals:

Define Clear Objectives: Set realistic and achievable goals that align with your overall health and fitness aspirations. Clearly defined objectives provide direction and motivation.

Break Down Goals: Break larger goals into smaller, actionable steps. This makes progress more tangible and helps you stay focused on achievable milestones.

Build a Support System:

Share Your Journey: Communicate your carb cycling journey with friends, family, or a community. Having a support system can provide encouragement, accountability, and understanding during challenges.

Seek Like-Minded Individuals: Connect with others who are also following a carb cycling approach.
Sharing experiences, recipes, and tips can foster a sense of community and motivation.

Track Progress:

Use Multiple Metrics: Beyond the scale, track various metrics such as body measurements, photos, and performance improvements. A holistic view of progress enhances motivation.

Regular Assessments: Conduct regular assessments to evaluate how your body responds to carb cycling. Adjust your approach based on these insights to optimize results.

Incorporate Flexibility:

Allow for Treats: Incorporate flexibility in your approach by allowing occasional treats. Allowing your-self to enjoy favorite foods in moderation reduces the likelihood of feeling deprived.

Adjust to Life Changes: Recognize that life is dynamic, and circumstances may change. Be flexible in adjusting your carb cycling approach to suit evolving needs.

Mindful Eating Practices:

Practice Mindfulness: Be present and mindful during meals. Pay attention to hunger and fullness cues, savor each bite, and appreciate the nourishment your meals provide.

Avoid Emotional Eating: Develop awareness of emotional triggers for eating. Implement strategies like deep breathing or engaging in a non-food-related activity when faced with emotional eating tendencies.

Educate Yourself:

Understand Nutrition: Continuously educate yourself about nutrition, macronutrients, and the science behind carb cycling. Knowledge empowers you to make informed choices and adapt your approach as needed.

Experiment with Foods: Explore a variety of foods to keep your meals interesting and enjoyable. Experimenting with recipes and ingredients prevents monotony and supports long-term adherence.

Celebrate Milestones:

Acknowledge Achievements: Celebrate your achievements along the way, whether they're related to fitness, improved energy levels, or adherence to your carb cycling plan.

Reward System: Establish a reward system for reaching milestones. Treat yourself to a non-food related reward, reinforcing positive behavior.

Staying consistent with carb cycling involves a combination of planning, flexibility, and mindfulness. By adopting these practices, you'll create a sustainable and enjoyable carb cycling journey that aligns with your health and fitness goals.

CHAPTER 11: TAILORING CARB CYCLING TO INDIVIDUAL NEEDS

Adapting Carb Cycling for Specific Health Conditions

One of the unique aspects of carb cycling is its flexibility, allowing individuals to tailor the approach to their specific health conditions. Whether managing diabetes, thyroid issues, or other health concerns, adapting carb cycling can be a valuable tool. Here's how to customize carb cycling to address specific health conditions:

Managing Diabetes:

Understanding Carbohydrate Impact: Individuals with diabetes need to carefully manage their carbohydrate intake to control blood sugar levels. When carb cycling, it's crucial to choose carbohydrates with a low glycemic index on low carb days. This includes whole grains, non-starchy vegetables, and legumes.

Regular Monitoring: Regularly monitor blood sugar levels to understand how different carb cycling phases impact your body. This helps in making informed adjustments to your carb intake based on your unique response.

Consulting Healthcare Professionals: Before implementing carb cycling, especially for those with diabetes, it's essential to consult with healthcare professionals, including a registered dietitian or endocrinologist. They can provide personalized guidance and ensure that the approach aligns with your diabetes management plan.

Thyroid Conditions:

Balancing Macronutrients: Individuals with thyroid conditions, such as hypothyroidism, may experience changes in metabolism. When carb cycling, ensure a balanced intake of macronutrients to support overall thyroid function. Adequate protein and healthy fats are essential for thyroid health.

Incorporating Selenium-Rich Foods: Selenium is a vital mineral for thyroid function. Consider incorporating selenium-rich foods such as Brazil nuts, fish, and sunflower seeds into your diet. Be mindful of your selenium intake, as excessive amounts can have adverse effects.

Consulting with Healthcare Providers: Those with thyroid conditions should consult with their healthcare providers, including an endocrinologist or nutritionist. Adjusting carb cycling based on individual thyroid health and medication requirements is crucial for optimal results.

Gut Health Concerns:

Emphasizing Fiber-Rich Foods: For individuals with gut health concerns, such as irritable bowel syndrome (IBS) or inflammatory bowel disease (IBD), carb cycling can be adjusted to emphasize fiber-rich foods that are gentle on the digestive system. This includes cooked vegetables, well-cooked grains, and easily digestible proteins.

Limiting Certain Foods: Some individuals with gut health concerns may need to limit specific types of carbohydrates, such as those high in FODMAPs (fermentable oligosaccharides, disaccharides, monosaccharides, and polyols). Adjusting carb cycling to include lower FODMAP options can be beneficial.

Professional Guidance: Seek guidance from healthcare professionals, including gastroenterologists or registered dietitians specializing in gut health. They can provide personalized advice on adapting carb cycling to support digestive well-being.

Cardiovascular Health:

Prioritizing Heart-Healthy Fats: Individuals with cardiovascular concerns can tailor carb cycling by prioritizing heart-healthy fats. This includes incorporating sources of omega3 fatty acids, such as fatty fish, flaxseeds, and walnuts, to support cardiovascular health.

Balancing Sodium Intake: Manage sodium intake, especially on high carb days, by choosing whole, minimally processed foods. Opt for fresh fruits, vegetables, and lean proteins to support a heart-healthy diet.

Regular Monitoring and Medical Consultation: Regularly monitor blood pressure and cholesterol levels. Consult with healthcare providers, including cardiologists and nutritionists, to ensure that carb cycling aligns with cardiovascular health goals.

Adapting carb cycling for specific health conditions requires a nuanced approach and collaboration with healthcare professionals. It emphasizes the importance of individualized dietary plans that consider the unique needs and challenges associated with different health conditions.

Customizing the Plan Based on Lifestyle and Preferences

One of the strengths of carb cycling lies in its adaptability to various lifestyles and individual preferences. Customizing the plan ensures that it aligns seamlessly with your daily routine and dietary choices. Here's how to tailor carb cycling to suit your lifestyle and preferences:

Busy Lifestyles:

Meal Prep and Planning: Individuals with hectic schedules can benefit from dedicated meal prep and planning. Prepare meals in advance, focusing on simplicity and efficiency. Batch cooking on designated days can save time throughout the week.

Portable Snack Options: Keep portable, nutrient-dense snacks on hand for busy days. Nuts, seeds, Greek yogurt, and pre-cut vegetables with hummus are convenient choices that align with carb cycling goals.

Flexible Scheduling: Adapt carb cycling to fit your schedule. Consider scheduling high carb days on days with more demanding activities or workouts, allowing for increased energy levels.

Vegetarian or Vegan Lifestyles:

Plant-Based Protein Sources: For those following vegetarian or vegan lifestyles, prioritize plant-based protein sources. Legumes, tofu, tempeh, quinoa, and a variety of nuts and seeds can be incorporated to meet protein needs.

Balancing Macronutrients: Ensure a balanced intake of macronutrients, especially protein, on all carb cycling days. Plant-based protein options can be combined with a mix of complex carbohydrates and healthy fats for a well-rounded approach.

Supplementation Considerations: Depending on individual nutritional needs, consider supplementing with vitamins and minerals commonly found in animal products, such as vitamin B12, iron, and omega3 fatty acids.

Intermittent Fasting:

Aligning with Fasting Windows: For those practicing intermittent fasting, tailor carb cycling to align with fasting windows. Schedule low carb days during fasting periods and high carb days during eating windows.

Strategic Meal Timing: Emphasize strategic meal timing to maximize the benefits of intermittent fasting. Consuming high carb meals post-workout during eating windows can support energy replenishment.

Hydration Focus: During fasting periods, prioritize hydration. Water, herbal teas, and other noncaloric beverages can help maintain hydration levels without breaking the fast.

Family and Social Commitments:

Flexible Planning: Carb cycling can be adapted to accommodate family meals and social gatherings. Plan high carb days on occasions when communal meals are central, allowing for enjoyment without compromising goals.

Communication and Support: Communicate your dietary preferences and goals with family and friends. Seek their support and understanding, fostering an environment that aligns with your carb cycling journey.

Smart Restaurant Choices: When dining out, make smart choices by selecting meals that align with the day's carb cycling phase. Many restaurants offer customizable options that cater to various dietary preferences.

Food Preferences:

Variety and Enjoyment: Incorporate a variety of foods to keep meals interesting and enjoyable. Experiment with different recipes, flavors, and cooking techniques to discover what aligns with your preferences.

Alternative Carb Sources: Explore alternative carb sources beyond traditional grains. Sweet potatoes, legumes, fruits, and root vegetables offer diverse options to suit different tastes.

Individualized Approach: Carb cycling allows for an individualized approach to food preferences. Whether you lean toward a Mediterranean, Asian, or plant-based diet, customize your carb cycling plan to embrace the foods you love.

CHAPTER 12: LONG-TERM SUCCESS AND MAINTENANCE

Strategies for Sustainable Nutrition

Sustainable nutrition is the cornerstone of long-term success in any dietary approach, including carb cycling. It goes beyond short-term goals, focusing on habits that can be maintained over time. Here are key strategies for ensuring sustainable nutrition:

Embrace Balanced Eating:

Diverse Nutrient Intake: Prioritize a diverse intake of nutrients by incorporating a variety of fruits, vegetables, lean proteins, whole grains, and healthy fats into your meals. This not only ensures adequate nutrition but also adds flavor and excitement to your diet.

Moderation and Portion Control: Practice moderation in your food choices and pay attention to portion sizes. Learning to recognize and respond to hunger and fullness cues contributes to a balanced and sustainable approach to eating.

Include Foods You Enjoy:

Indulge in Moderation: Depriving yourself of foods you enjoy can lead to feelings of restriction. Allow yourself to indulge in favorite foods in moderation, even on low carb days. This flexibility fosters a positive relationship with food.

Explore Healthy Alternatives: Find healthier alternatives for your favorite dishes. Experiment with recipes that use whole, nutrient-dense ingredients while still capturing the flavors you love. This way, you can enjoy your meals without compromising nutritional goals.

Gradual and Mindful Changes:

Slow Implementation: Implement changes gradually to allow for adaptation. Abrupt and drastic shifts in eating habits are often challenging to sustain. Gradual adjustments make it easier to adopt new habits over time.

Mindful Eating Practices: Practice mindful eating by savoring each bite, eating without distractions, and paying attention to hunger and fullness signals. This mindful approach enhances the overall dining experience and promotes sustainable habits.

Educate Yourself:

Continuous Learning: Stay informed about nutrition, macronutrients, and the science behind carb cycling. Continuous learning empowers you to make informed choices, adapt your approach based on evolving knowledge, and navigate nutritional information with confidence.

Experiment and Adjust: As you educate yourself, be open to experimenting with different approaches. Your nutritional needs may evolve over time, and being adaptable allows you to make informed adjustments to your carb cycling plan.

Build a Support System:

Community and Accountability: Connect with others who share similar dietary goals. Building a support system provides a sense of community, accountability, and encouragement. Share experiences, challenges, and successes to stay motivated.

Involve Family and Friends: Engage your family and friends in your journey towards sustainable nutrition. Encourage shared meals and involve them in the preparation of carb cycling friendly dishes. Creating a supportive environment positively influences long-term success.

Monitoring Progress and Adjusting the Plan

Monitoring progress and making adjustments to your carb cycling plan are integral components of long-term success. Regular assessments allow you to stay on track and refine your approach as needed.

Here's how to effectively monitor progress and make informed adjustments:

Regular Assessments:

Scale and Beyond: While the scale is a useful tool, rely on a combination of metrics to assess progress. Include measurements, photos, changes in energy levels, and improvements in performance to get a holistic view of your journey.

Consistent Tracking: Establish a consistent tracking system to monitor changes over time. Whether it's a weekly check-in or a monthly assessment, regular tracking helps identify patterns and trends.

Evaluate Energy Levels:

Subjective Feelings: Pay attention to subjective feelings of energy and vitality. Improved energy levels are often indicators of a well-balanced and effective carb cycling approach. Conversely, persistent fatigue may signal a need for adjustments.

Performance in Workouts: Assess your performance in workouts as an additional measure of progress. Increased strength, endurance, and overall performance can indicate that your nutritional plan is supporting your fitness goals.

Adjust Based on Goals:

Reassess Goals Periodically: Goals may evolve over time, and periodic reassessment is crucial. Whether your focus shifts from weight loss to muscle building or vice versa, adjust your carb cycling plan to align with your current objectives.

Tailor Carb Cycling Phases: Modify the distribution of low, moderate, and high carb days based on your evolving goals. For example, if muscle building becomes a priority, consider adjusting the frequency and timing of high carb days to support increased energy demands.

Listen to Your Body:

Hunger and Satiety Cues: Tune in to your body's hunger and satiety cues. If you consistently feel overly restricted or uncomfortably full, consider adjusting your macronutrient ratios or the timing of your meals to better suit your individual needs.

Individual Responses: Recognize that everyone's body responds differently to carb cycling. Experiment with variations and observe how your body reacts. Being attuned to individual responses allows for a more personalized and effective approach.

Professional Guidance:

Consult with Experts: Seek guidance from healthcare professionals, nutritionists, or fitness experts when needed. If progress stalls or you encounter challenges, consulting with professionals can provide valuable insights and recommendations.

Nutritional Counseling: Consider nutritional counseling to receive personalized advice based on your unique needs and goals. A registered dietitian can offer tailored strategies to optimize your carb cycling plan for long-term success.

Lifestyle Changes for Overall Well-being

Achieving long-term success with carb cycling extends beyond dietary adjustments. Implementing lifestyle changes that enhance overall well-being contributes to sustained health and fitness. Here are key lifestyle changes that complement your carb cycling journey:

Regular Physical Activity:

Incorporate Exercise: Physical activity is a crucial component of overall well-being. Incorporate a mix of cardiovascular exercise, strength training, and flexibility exercises into your routine. Tailor your workouts to align with your fitness goals and energy levels.

Consistent Routine: Establish a consistent exercise routine. Whether it's morning walks, gym sessions, or home workouts, regular physical activity contributes to improved mood, energy levels, and overall health.

Adequate Sleep:

Prioritize Sleep: Quality sleep is essential for recovery, energy levels, and overall health. Prioritize consistent sleep patterns, create a conducive sleep environment, and aim for the recommended seven to nine hours of sleep per night.

Establish a Routine: Establish a bedtime routine to signal to your body that it's time to wind down. Limit screen time before bed, create a comfortable sleep environment, and engage in relaxing activities such as reading or gentle stretching.

Stress Management:

Mindfulness Practices: Incorporate mindfulness practices into your daily routine. Techniques such as meditation, deep breathing, or yoga can help manage stress levels and promote a sense of calm.

Identify Stressors: Identify and address sources of stress in your life. Whether through lifestyle adjustments, setting boundaries, or seeking support, managing stress positively impacts both mental and physical wellbeing.

Hydration:

Consistent Water Intake: Stay consistently hydrated by drinking an adequate amount of water throughout the day. Proper hydration supports digestion, energy levels, and overall health.

Hydrating Foods: Include hydrating foods in your diet, such as fruits and vegetables with high water content.

These contribute to overall hydration and provide essential vitamins and minerals.

CHAPTER 13: SUCCESS STORIES AND TESTIMONIES

Success Stories and Testimonials: Real-Life
Experiences of Women Over50 with Carb Cycling

Embarking on a health and fitness journey, especially one as nuanced as carb cycling, can be both challenging and rewarding. In this chapter, we delve into the inspiring success stories and testimonials of women over 50 who have embraced carb cycling as a lifestyle. These narratives offer valuable insights, motivation, and practical tips for anyone considering or already navigating the path of carb cycling.

Inspiration for Overcoming Challenges
and Achieving Goals

Jane's Transformation Journey:

Jane, a 55-year-old woman, began her carb cycling journey as a means to break through a weight loss plateau. Despite regular exercise, her progress had stagnated, and she sought a sustainable approach that would align with her age and hormonal changes.

Initially, Jane encountered challenges in adapting to low carb days. She experienced fluctuations in energy levels and occasional cravings. However, her determination and the support of a carb cycling community kept her motivated.

Over time, Jane noticed significant improvements in her body composition. She shed excess body fat, gained lean muscle, and felt a renewed sense of vitality. Jane's story exemplifies the power of perseverance and the positive impact of carb cycling on both physical and mental wellbeing.

Sarah's Menopausal Journey:

Sarah, at 52, faced the challenges of menopause, including weight gain and hormonal fluctuations. Frustrated by traditional dieting methods, she turned to carb cycling as a way to navigate the unique aspects of nutrition during this life stage.

Sarah tailored her carb cycling plan to accommodate the hormonal changes associated with menopause. She strategically included foods that supported hormonal balance, such as flaxseeds and cruciferous vegetables, and found that carb cycling helped manage symptoms like hot flashes.

Sarah's success extends beyond weight management. She reports enhanced mental clarity, improved sleep quality, and increased energy levels. Her journey highlights the importance of recognizing and adapting nutrition to align with the specific challenges of menopause.

Grace's Active Lifestyle:

Grace, a 58-year-old fitness enthusiast, incorporated carb cycling to optimize her performance and recovery. Her primary goal was to maintain an active lifestyle and ensure that her nutritional choices supported her fitness endeavors.

Grace strategically timed high carb days around her most intense workout sessions. This approach provided the necessary energy for challenging workouts and facilitated better recovery.

By aligning her nutrition with her fitness goals, Grace not only sustained her active lifestyle but also noticed improvements in her overall strength and endurance. Her experience demonstrates how carb cycling can be tailored to meet the specific needs of individuals with active lifestyles.

Key Themes from Success Stories:

Adaptability for Life Stages: Carb cycling proved adaptable to various life stages, including menopause and post-menopausal years. Women found success by adjusting their nutritional approach to align with hormonal changes, demonstrating that carb cycling can be a supportive tool during different phases of life.

Improved Hormonal Balance:

Several testimonials highlighted improvements in hormonal balance. Whether managing menopausal symptoms or addressing hormonal fluctuations, women reported positive changes, emphasizing the potential benefits of carb cycling for hormonal health.

Enhanced Mental Clarity and Energy:

Mental well-being and increased energy levels were common themes. Women noted improvements in mental clarity, focus, and sustained energy throughout the day, showcasing the broader impact of carb cycling on overall vitality.

Personalized Fitness Support:

Tailoring carb cycling to support fitness goals emerged as a recurring theme. Whether pursuing weight training, cardiovascular exercise, or a combination of activities, women found success by strategically incorporating high carb days to optimize performance and recovery.

CONCLUSION

One of the central advantages of carb cycling for women over 50 lies in its ability to optimize fat burning while preserving lean muscle mass. The cyclical nature of this approach accommodates the body's changing needs, providing essential nutrients during high carb days and tapping into fat stores during low carb periods. This not only aids in weight loss but also contributes to maintaining muscle mass, a crucial aspect for overall health and vitality carb cycling emerges as a valuable and viable strategy for women over 50 in their pursuit of sustainable weight management and overall health. By understanding the science, customizing the approach to individual needs, and navigating challenges with practical solutions, carb cycling becomes more than a dietary strategy —it transforms into a lifestyle choice that empowers women over 50 to embrace wellness with vitality and enthusiasm.

Made in United States
Orlando, FL
04 August 2024

49907319R00067